JOHN MUIR TRAIL
The essential guide to hiking America's most famous trail

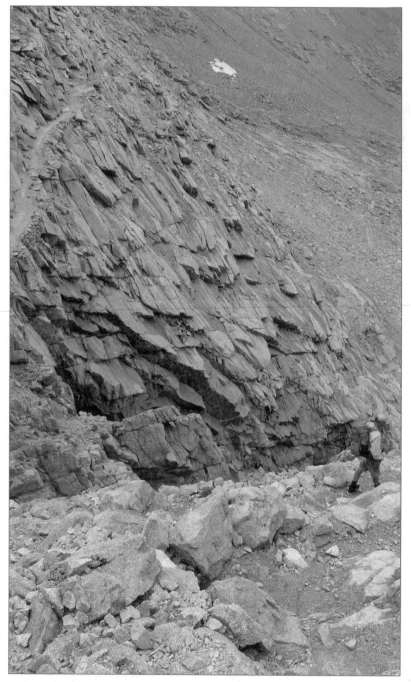

Descending the switchbacks on the south side of Forester Pass

JOHN MUIR TRAIL
The essential guide to hiking America's most famous trail

Elizabeth Wenk

 WILDERNESS PRESS ... *on the trail since 1967*

John Muir Trail: The essential guide to hiking America's most famous trail

5th Edition
  2nd printing 2015
Copyright © 1978, 1984, 1998, 2007, 2014 by Wilderness Press
Front and back cover photos copyright © 2014 by Elizabeth Wenk
Unless otherwise noted, all interior photos by Elizabeth Wenk
Maps: Elizabeth Wenk
Cover design: Scott McGrew
Editor: Amber Kaye Henderson

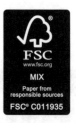

ISBN: 978-0-89997-736-2; eISBN: 978-0-89997-737-9
Manufactured in the United States of America

Published by: **Wilderness Press**
             c/o Keen Communications
             PO Box 43673
             Birmingham, AL 35243
             800-443-7227; FAX 205-326-1012
             wildernesspress.com

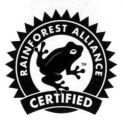

Visit our website for a complete listing of our books and for ordering information.

Distributed by Publishers Group West

Front cover, clockwise from top left: Donohue Pass Trail, Garnet Lake, and the Golden Staircase; *Back cover, top to bottom:* North side of Island Pass and Silver Pass Creek

SAFETY NOTICE: Although Wilderness Press and the author have made every attempt to ensure that the information in this book is accurate at press time, they are not responsible for any loss, damage, injury, or inconvenience that may occur to anyone while using this book. You are responsible for your own safety and health while in the wilderness. The fact that a trail is described in this book does not mean that it will be safe for you. Be aware that trail conditions can change from day to day. Always check local conditions and know your own limitations.

CONTENTS

LIST OF MAPS

ACKNOWLEDGMENTS

While only short stretches of California's John Muir Trail (JMT) have been rerouted in the seven years since the fourth edition of this book was published in 2007, a trail guide nevertheless requires updating, both to accurately represent the continually changing landscape and to reflect modern thinking and trends. For me that required not just rehiking the JMT, but also extensive consultation with others; their knowledge and perspectives have made this book much richer.

I am especially appreciative of the interactions I have had with National Park Service staff, including Naomi Chakrin, George Durkee, Greg Fauth, David Gordon, Chris Miles, Martijn Ouborg, Rob Pilewski, Alison Steiner, Jen VanDragt, and Ken Watson. As the JMT continues to grow in popularity, hikers increasingly impact the stripe of wilderness through which the trail passes, and it is important to me to consult with the local "rangers" (broadly speaking) to minimize the impact. They spent time reviewing key information provided in the book and discussing their experiences with me. I thank them enormously for this input.

I would also like to thank the many hikers whom I met on the trail this summer for their conversation and insights. Hiking a long trail is about more than covering the miles and seeing the scenery: it is also about the other people who are sharing the same experience, each through their own lens. I thoroughly enjoyed listening to others' experiences and did my best to weave their suggestions into this next edition.

Many scientists fact-checked sections of the book. Robert Derlett, professor of medicine at the University of California, Davis researches High Sierra water quality and read through my text on water quality and treatment; Greg Stock, the Yosemite National Park geologist, read through the geologic information included in the book; Roland Knapp, a researcher at the Sierra Nevada Aquatic Research Lab, reviewed the information about the mountain yellow-legged frogs; and John Wehausen, a researcher at the White Mountain Research Station, read through my text on large mammals. In addition to the time they spent reading my manuscript, I am grateful for the time they, and others, have spent learning ever more about the Sierra, for in-depth knowledge of the ecosystem's natural history enriches the hike for all of us.

One of the most time-consuming additions to this edition are my own topo maps, for which I intended to use GPS tracks I had collected for both the John Muir Trail and all of the major access trails over the past few years. Here technology thwarted my best efforts, as my primary GPS corrupted and deleted some of my data on several days this past summer. I therefore need to acknowledge other hikers who generously provided their own GPS tracks for trails where I lost my data or which I could not visit in the past few summers. Many thanks to David Harris, Seth Heringer, Joerg Lohse, Dave Lubertozzi, and Matt Maxon.

And most important I need to thank my family and friends with whom I hiked and who made this hike possible. As a mother of two young daughters, Eleanor and Sophia, disappearing into the mountains for a month required the support and help of many others, especially my mother, Julia, and husband, Douglas. But I also applaud Eleanor and Sophia as well as their cousins Jane and Liam, whose small legs trudged slowly from Tuolumne Meadows to Agnew Meadows. And two friends, Tara Cameron and Steve Jones, provided wonderful companionship along the middle 100-mile stretch of the JMT.

—Elizabeth Wenk
Sydney, Australia, March 2014

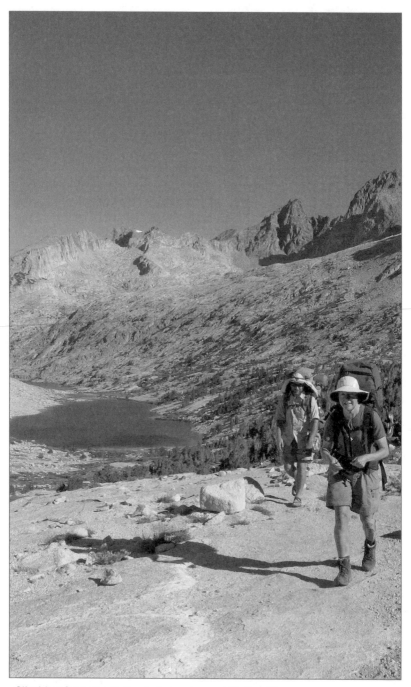

Climbing from the Palisade Lakes toward Mather Pass

INTRODUCTION

The John Muir Trail (or, more simply, the JMT) passes through what many backpackers agree is the finest mountain scenery in the United States. Some hikers may give first prize to some other place, but none will deny the great attractiveness of California's High Sierra. This is a land of 13,000- and 14,000-foot peaks, of soaring granite cliffs, of lakes by the thousands, and of canyons 5,000 feet deep. It is a land where trails touch only a tiny portion of the total area, so that by leaving the path, you can find utter solitude. It is a land uncrossed by road for 140 miles as the crow flies, from Sherman Pass in the south to Tioga Pass in the north. And perhaps best of all, it is a land blessed with the mildest, sunniest climate of any major mountain range in the world. Though rain does fall in the summer—as does much snow in the winter—it seldom lasts more than an hour or two, and the sun is out and shining most of the hours of the day. You are, of course, not the only person to have heard of these attractions and will encounter people daily, but the trail really is a thin line through a vast land; with little effort you can always camp on your own if you leave the trail.

This book describes the JMT from its northern terminus at Happy Isles to its southern terminus atop Mt. Whitney, and then to Whitney Portal, the nearest trailhead, for a total of 220 miles of magnificent Sierra scenery. For those who prefer to walk south to north, a description written in reverse is available in a separate electronic version of the book. The book is aimed at all hikers: hikers completing the entire JMT in a single trip, as well as those walking a shorter section of the trail; hikers completing the route in 10 days and those taking a month. As a result, the guide does not include suggested daily itineraries, as each person or group has a different pace, different desires for layover days, lazy afternoons around camp, or detours to nearby peaks or lake basins. Instead, this guide is aimed to provide you with

1

background knowledge and let you design your own trip, in advance or as you walk. The book provides information on distances, lateral trails, established camping locations, notable stream crossings, long climbs, especially splendid lakes, detours up worthy peaks, and a bit of natural history to encourage you to gaze at your surroundings. From there, you design the itinerary that best suits you.

Finally, one thought to carry on your walk: The nature of the High Sierra changes dramatically from north to south, and often from one mile to the next. With each step, enjoy and absorb where you are, rather than comparing it with where you have been or where you are headed. The grandeur and relief of the southern regions are undeniably striking, but there is no reason to expect (or desire) your entire journey to look like the headwaters of the Kern; if you did, you would spend three weeks sitting atop Bighorn Plateau. Instead, by hiking the length of the High Sierra, you are choosing to embrace the variation in landscape, topography, geology, biology, weather, and more. Could you possibly compare the domes of Tuolumne Meadows, the volcanic landscape near Devils Postpile, the dense stands of mountain hemlocks north of Silver Pass, the lakes of Evolution Basin, the foxtail pines on Bighorn Plateau, or the view from the summit of Mt. Whitney? By the end of your walk, you likely will comment that they are all fantastic and memorable, each in its own way. If a section of the landscape doesn't grab you, watch a nearby stream tumble over boulders, stare at the plants by your feet, follow the sound of the birdcalls to the treetops, or look at the minerals in a rock. These are all part of the continually changing landscape of the magnificent High Sierra.

Using This Book

The trail description is split into 13 sections, one for each of the river drainages through which the JMT passes. While you are often confined to a single watershed on a shorter walk, part of the glory of the JMT is that you can see how the landscape changes between drainages. Each section begins with a detailed elevation profile of the trail. Marked on the elevation profile are most of the junctions you will pass. Campsites are shown on the topo maps, with more detailed descriptions provided in Appendix B.

Also included at the beginning of each trail section is a table listing the major junctions you will pass, as well as some other waypoints. Each entry includes the elevation, UTM coordinates, distance from the previous point, and cumulative distance from the JMT endpoints, here given as Happy Isles and Whitney Portal. All elevations have been rounded to the closest 10 feet, as I do not believe my measurements from maps or from my GPS unit are more accurate than this—and possibly only half this good. The elevations of the major junctions and distances between these junctions are also indicated in the text using the following notation: [7,010' – 1.5/116.0]. This example lets you know that you are at an elevation of 7,010 feet, you have traveled 1.5 miles since the last junction noted, and you have traveled 116 miles since Happy Isles.

Following the tables is a written description taking you along the JMT. This covers trail conditions, river crossings, and camping areas, as well as some details of the vegetation communities and geologic features you pass on your hike. (The text is not intended to be read as an adventure story before starting your journey, but rather during breaks as you hike along.) Note that all UTM coordinates given in this book follow the North American datum 1927, as this is the reference system used on most USGS 7.5-minute maps (as well as Tom Harrison's maps). GPS devices and mapping software packages use NAD 1983 as a default, but these can easily convert between the two reference systems.

Maps

The topographic maps within this book are derived from the latest digital elevation models available from the U.S. Geological Survey. I am pleasantly surprised that the topo lines generated from these new models match nearly perfectly with those shown on the decade-old USGS topos. Overlaid on these are layers with information on water bodies, roads, and geographic names, also courtesy of the USGS. As for the trails, the JMT and about 75% of the side trails shown are derived from GPS tracks that I have collected over the past few years. The route for the JMT was further corrected by editing it to match the latest aerial photos provided by ExpertGPS and Google Earth, allowing me to more accurately measure the distance where the trail has switchbacks; this added about a mile to my estimated length of the entire JMT. GPS tracks for a few additional side trails came from others who kindly shared tracks with me. The remaining side trails have been traced off USGS topo maps, as I was not carrying a GPS when I most recently hiked them; research on my part indicates that the total trail length is rarely more than 5% different between the actual track and what is approximated on the USGS topo maps, although the actual route often deviates in sections.

(Continued on page 6)

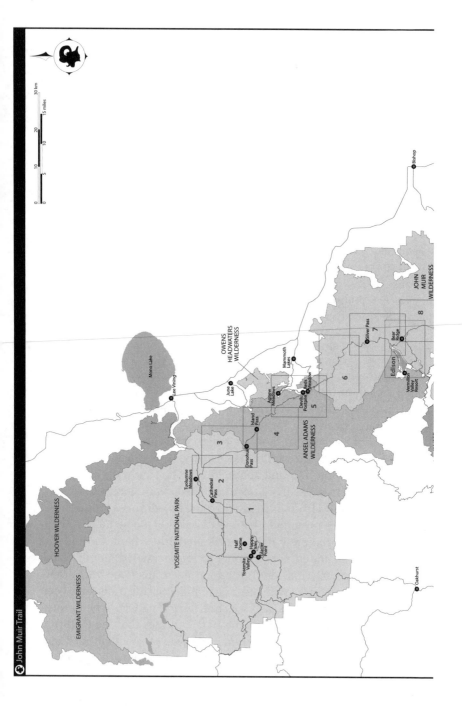

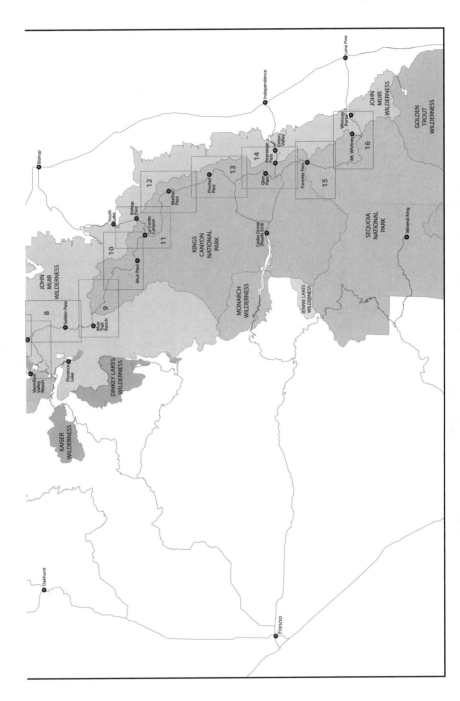

(Continued from page 3)

If you wish to supplement these maps with a second map, a popular choice are Tom Harrison's JMT map pack or his individual "High Sierra" maps for different regions along the JMT. I am still very fond of the traditional USGS 7.5-minute topo maps, but acknowledge that they are heavy, becoming difficult to purchase, and contain an unnecessary level of detail if you are only hiking on trails.

People are increasingly carrying maps on a range of digital devices; search for "John Muir Trail digital maps" for the current selection. However, I urge you to carry some paper map with you, for digital devices are unreliable. I have encountered multiple people with broken devices or insufficient batteries who have found themselves on the trail without a map (or other trail information). Even for data collection I carry two GPS units, after both friends and I have repeatedly had devices fail.

Note that a derivative of this book, *John Muir Trail Data Book,* is also available. It contains the same tables and maps as this book but lacks the background information and trail description.

An electronic version of the UTM coordinates is available as a file at **groups.yahoo.com/neo/groups/johnmuirtrail/info.**

Map Legend

Symbol	Description	Symbol	Description
●	JMT junction	———	John Muir Trail
▲7.08	JMT campsite	··········	Maintained trail
⌂	Ranger station	········	Unmaintained trail
▲	Summit	═══	Road (paved)
)(	Pass	=======	Road (unpaved)
	Body of water	· — · — · ·	National park or forest boundary
	Glacier or permanent snowfield	– – – –	Wilderness boundary
⩘	Marsh	⌄2000–	index contours 1000 feet
———	Stream		(contour interval 200 feet)
∧∧∧∧∧∧∧∧	Ridgeline	⇡	magnetic north 13°05' east of geographic north
⫱⫱⫱⫱⫱⫱⫱	Cliffs		1927 North American datum

PLANNING YOUR HIKE

You should not embark on the John Muir Trail on impulse. Its length, remoteness, altitude, and continuous ascents and descents mean that you must plan your hike and know what to expect if you are going to enjoy it.

First, you need sufficient backpacking experience to know how your appetite behaves on long hikes, how much your body can take without rebelling, and especially how your emotions react in various backpacking situations. For example, you will have your own typical reactions to solitude (if you go alone), forced togetherness (if you don't go alone), cold, heat, rain, excessive mosquitoes, and injury.

Second, it is helpful to know a bit about backpacking in the Sierra to gauge your expected progress. If this is your first time here, consider the following: the general lack of lousy weather means that you can plan to hike for as many hours as your body will take. With few exceptions, the JMT is well-graded with numerous switchbacks easing the long climbs; rocky trails over passes and through some high basins can be hard on your feet, limiting daily mileage; and much of the trail is at high altitude, slowing progress.

Given these parameters, most JMT hikers cover 10–12 miles per day, although in this era of ultralight gear (and short vacations), there are ever more people ticking off 16–20, or more, miles each day. I advocate hiking no more than 15 miles per day and setting aside a handful of layover (or zero) days, for there are so many beautiful scenes to absorb and so many side trails, lakes, or peaks to explore (see the chapter beginning on page 209 for suggestions). It is especially nice to have the flexibility of stopping early on a day you feel beat, so you can enjoy the upcoming stretch of trail with a fresh body in the morning. I am amazed how fatigue or a bad attitude can color my perception of trail segments; when I feel worse, I find that the scenery escapes my notice and I spend the walk wanting to reach the next junction instead of reveling in the location's beauty. If you find that you walk faster or farther than you anticipate, and have extra time, you can always explore a nearby peak or spend a relaxing afternoon in a picturesque location. To estimate how many days the JMT will take you to hike, divide 220.8 (the total overall mileage) by your expected daily mileage. Add the number of 0-mile days you would like to take, and you have the total elapsed days. Using the cumulative mileage table, beginning on page 62, and the campsite list (Appendix B), you can pick tentative destinations for each night.

Some hikers prefer to hike the trail in one- or two-week legs, spread over more than one season. This book will help you do that: Appendix A describes the lateral trails used to access the JMT, how to reach each of the trailheads from the nearest town, and how to obtain permits. Other Wilderness Press publications, including *Sierra North*, *Sierra South*, and *Sequoia & Kings Canyon National Parks*, provide greater detail on these lateral trails.

North to South, or South to North?

Although the trail was scouted north to south, south to north was for many years the preferred direction to hike the JMT. Today, however, rangers estimate that somewhere between 90% to 96% of hikers are headed in the opposite direction, from Yosemite Valley to Mt. Whitney. All hikers I queried were enjoying their chosen direction—and most felt strongly that it was the preferable direction. I took away from my survey that, as expected, everyone hiking the JMT is having a good time and would still be enjoying him- or herself if walking in the opposite direction. Nonetheless, I have listed below some reasons why people advocated a given direction of travel:

Some reasons for hiking south to north include:
- The sun is not in your eyes as you walk.
- If your trip is cut short, you have had a chance to see the most dramatic mountain landscape.
- Climbing 6,000 feet out of Yosemite Valley in midsummer is miserably hot.
- You are headed the same direction as PCT hikers and can relate to their trail tales.
- It is the classic direction.

Some reasons for hiking north to south include:
- You do not have to put up with the Mt. Whitney permit lottery.

- Your uphills are mostly north-facing and therefore more forested and shadier.
- You are better acclimated by the time you hit the high passes, not to mention Mt. Whitney.
- The scenery just keeps getting more dramatic as you head south.
- Because most people are headed the same direction as you, you will see fewer people as you walk.
- This is the direction that the trail was first scouted.

Because the vast majority of today's hikers are southbound, the print version of this edition only includes the southbound trail descriptions. However, the northbound description is available in a separate electronic edition.

When Should You Go?

Several factors, including temperature, snow cover, stream crossings, mosquitoes, flowers, and the number of people on the trail, may influence your decision about when to hike the JMT. Each person will, of course, have his or her own opinion on which of these should set the exact departure date. However, one factor trumps all others, such that nearly everyone embarks on the trail sometime between early July and mid-September, for it is during these months that you are guaranteed mostly snow-free travel.

Temperatures will be warmest in July and early August. On average, snow cover will be minimal by early to mid-July, but due to enormous variation year to year, there is no normal year, only average snowfall quantities. In big snow years, most of the upper elevations will be covered in snow through mid-July, making progress much slower and more arduous. (Additional information on temperatures and snow cover can be found in the weather section beginning on page 38.) Stream levels are strongly correlated with snow cover, such that during late June and early July, on average, stream levels will be very high and crossing can be dangerous. Mosquitoes are likewise unpredictable, but they tend to be terrible in early July, tolerable by late July or early August, and nearly absent following the first cold nights in mid-August. The period of the peak flower bloom, unfortunately, lags the mosquitoes by only a week, with the most spectacular displays in mid-July. As the peak flow of people tends to be mid-July—late August, some hikers choose to begin their trips after Labor Day (early September) to experience greater solitude on the trail. The first light snowfalls tend to occur during

September, but usually melt quickly, while mid- to late October often brings the first larger storms that abruptly end the backpacking season and cause trouble for parties deep in the wilderness.

Gear and Supplies

If this will be your longest wilderness trip ever, I recommend that you glance through a how-to-backpack book (such as Brian Beffort's *Joy of Backpacking*, also published by Wilderness Press), as well as some online trip reports from other people hiking the JMT. The John Muir Trail forum on Yahoo Groups is an inviting place to ask questions and also hosts a large collection of help sheets. Raymond E. Rippel's **jmtbook.com** is another good resource. From such sources you should devise your own checklist of essential equipment, including gear you deem necessary for comfort or safety, and probably a few extras that will enhance your trip, such as a camera and a copy of this book. If you have purchased new equipment for your trek, be sure to test it before discovering its shortcomings on the first day of your long-planned vacation.

Both your gear list and the weight of each item make an enormous difference to your base pack weight—and that is weight that you will carry for 220.8 miles—so think hard about your gear decisions. *Ultralight Backpackin' Tips* by Mike Clelland (Falcon Guides, 2011) offers plenty of ideas on how to reduce weight. Some of these will make sense to you, while others may seem too minimalist, but reading through it does force you to think about what you are planning to pack.

One of the most divisive gear questions is what footwear is appropriate. After many discussions (arguments?) with friends over the correct shoes to wear on a trip, I've come to the conclusion that most options are "correct," but that each person needs to know his or her preference in advance of a long trip. On one hike down the JMT, I wore mountaineering boots, and my husband wore running shoes. We were both very content (and compatible) hikers. His feet and knees would have constantly ached in heavy boots, and I would have twisted my ankles and had sore arches in less sturdy footwear.

In today's era of food-storage canisters (see page 31), backpacking food must be compact as well as lightweight. To maximize use of your bear canister, ditch extra packaging and repack any bulky items into small zip-top plastic bags. Many hikers opt for the freeze-dried backpacker foods, but with a little time, and much less money, you can create your own concoctions. Visit a local bulk food store to find a variety of quick-cooking grains and flavorings. You can likely find several backpacking cuisine books at your local outdoor store. One of my favorite meals is cranberries, cashews, powdered coconut milk, curry powder, and couscous. Bring the coconut milk and dried cranberries to a boil (with a little more water than the couscous requires), and then throw in the rest and turn off the stove.

If you are flying into California and must organize your food for the trip once you arrive here, the stores in Yosemite Valley and Tuolumne Meadows have a fairly good selection of food for backpacking trips and are acceptably priced. Alternatively, the towns of Bishop and Mammoth Lakes have large grocery stores and camping stores. If you are in the larger cities in western California, hunt for bulk food stores or visit Trader Joe's.

Emergency Beacons and Contacts

A recent addition to many packs is a type of emergency beacon (for example, a Personal Emergency Position-Indicating Radio Beacon [PEPIRB]) or a personal GPS tracking device (for example, a Spot device). Because cell phone coverage along the JMT is restricted to Tuolumne Meadows, Reds Meadow, a region around Lake Edison and Bear Ridge, and the summit of Mt. Whitney (and even then only with the right carrier), many people carry emergency beacons in case of an emergency or to send regular messages to family members. Research the choices and select what is best for you, but some words of warning: don't set it off if you can self-evacuate and don't imagine that by carrying it you can push yourself beyond your normal safe boundaries, which could inconvenience and endanger the rescuers, often volunteers. And while PEPIRBs are (nearly) assured to function, people have intermittent success with Spot devices.

Should you find yourself in an emergency situation, here are the numbers you need. Note that these are emergency only numbers—do not contact them for other questions!

EMERGENCY NUMBERS		
Jurisdiction	Trail sections	Phone numbers
Yosemite NP	1–2	209-379-1992
Madera County Sheriff	4	559-675-7770
Devils Postpile NM	4	760-934-2289
Fresno County Sheriff	5–7	559-488-3111 (use when outside Kings Canyon NP)
Sequoia and Kings Canyon NP	7–12	559-565-3195 or 559-565-3341
Inyo County Sheriff	3, 13	760-878-0395 or 760-878-0235

Wilderness Permits

All trailheads accessing the JMT require a wilderness permit and have quotas. For all Sierra wilderness areas, permits are issued for the trailhead and date at which you begin your hike. This single permit is valid for the entire length of your hike: you do not need to obtain a new permit either when you enter a new jurisdiction or when you exit the JMT to resupply. The one exception to this blanket rule is exiting via Mt. Whitney: the Inyo National Forest requires that all parties exiting via the Mt. Whitney Zone are subject to exit quotas (25 people per day). However, if you begin your trip outside of Inyo or Sierra National Forests, you are not subject to the exit quota. (*Note:* If you are on a longer trip in the western Sierra that does not exit over Trail Crest, you may hike up Mt. Whitney from the western slope without a permit.)

Appendix A lists most entry points to the JMT and identifies both the agency from which and the trailhead for which you must get a permit. The next page provides a timetable for permit reservations. This information is subject to change, but the enormous variation between agencies' "when, how, and cost" will probably always exist—don't wait until the last moment to check the agency's website. Throughout the summer season, the Yosemite National Park and Inyo National Forest websites also indicate on what days permits are still available for each trailhead. A word of warning: Quotas for reserved permits fill very quickly in summer. Reserve your permit as soon as they become available and, if possible, have alternate, weekday start dates as potential backups. Alternatively, plan to obtain a first-come, first-serve permit the day before, but again, plan on being at the permit station at—or before—the time you can first get a permit because they will disappear very fast. Obtaining permits to begin hikes at both Whitney Portal and Happy Isles is difficult. A number of southbound hikers choose to day hike from Yosemite Valley to Tuolumne (which does not require a permit) and then obtain a permit for Lyell Canyon to continue their walk. Others begin their walk at Glacier Point and join the JMT at the Panorama Trail junction, 2.8 miles from Happy Isles. Some northbound hikers begin at Cottonwood Pass or Cottonwood Lakes to the south of Whitney Portal.

Because most permits need to be picked up in person, you need to make sure that you are at a ranger station during business hours, usually 8 a.m.–5 p.m., daily. Permits for the Mt. Whitney Trail can only be picked up at the Eastern Sierra Interagency Visitor Center, a few miles south of Lone Pine, while other Inyo National Forest permits can be picked up at any of its ranger stations.

Permit Reservation Information

Agency	When to Reserve	How to Reserve	Cost	Percent of Permits Available for Reservation	First-Come, First-Serve Permit Availability
Yosemite NP	24 weeks in advance	Phone, mail, fax*	$5 per permit + $5 per person	60%	11 a.m. day before entry
Inyo NF	6 months in advance	Internet	$6 per permit + $5 per person**	60%	11 a.m., day before entry, but can fill in request form at 8 a.m.
Whitney Portal (Inyo NF)	February 1, by lottery	Internet	$15 per person	100%	Only cancellations available
Sierra NF	1 year in advance	Mail	$5 per person	60%	Wilderness station opening, day before entry
Sequoia/Kings Canyon NP	March 1	Mail, fax	$15 per group	75%	1 p.m., day before entry

* You can fax in permits after the office closes at 5 p.m. PST the day before. Applications received by this method are processed in random order at 8 a.m. the following morning.

** $15 per person if exiting at Whitney Portal

Permit Offices

Yosemite National Park Wilderness Permit Office
PO Box 545
Yosemite, CA 95389
209-372-0740 (Monday–Friday, 8:30 a.m.–4:30 p.m.)
nps.gov/yose/planyourvisit/wildpermits.htm
Note: If you begin your walk in Yosemite, you will most likely use one of three permits: Happy Isles to Little Yosemite Valley (if you plan to spend your first night at the Little Yosemite Valley campsite), Happy Isles to Sunrise/Merced Lake (pass-through; if you plan to spend your first night at the Clouds Rest junction or beyond), or Lyell Canyon (if you plan to begin your southbound hike in Tuolumne Meadows).

Inyo National Forest Wilderness Permit Offices
760-873-2485 (wilderness information)
recreation.gov (for reservations)
www.fs.usda.gov/inyo (look under Passes & Permits, then Recreation Passes
    & Permits for information)
Note: If you are departing from Whitney Portal, you will need a permit for the Mt. Whitney Trail, available only by a lottery held in February.

High Sierra Ranger District (Sierra National Forest)
Attn: Wilderness Permits
PO Box 559
Prather, CA 93651
559-855-5355 (wilderness information only; not for reservations)
tinyurl.com/sierrapermit

Sequoia and Kings Canyon National Parks
Wilderness Permit Reservations
47050 Generals Hwy. #60
Three Rivers, CA 93271
559-565-3766 (wilderness information only; not for reservations)
559-565-4239 (fax)
nps.gov/seki/planyourvisit/wilderness_permits.htm

Transportation

There are two separate transportation challenges you face hiking the
JMT: how to get to (and from) the Sierra (described first) and how to get
back to your car at the end of this trip. While California locals generally
opt to drive to the mountains, those arriving by air often prefer to use
public transport to get to (or from) the Sierra. The information on getting to the Sierra focuses on transport from the San Francisco Bay Area,
Los Angeles International Airport (LAX), and between towns once in
the Sierra. Others are flying to smaller airports, including Reno, Merced, Bakersfield, Fresno, Inyokern, that have connections to the same
public transit networks.

Getting to the Sierra by Public Transport

Flying directly to Mammoth Lakes The small Mammoth Yosemite
airport (MMH) is located just outside the town of Mammoth Lakes.
In summer there are currently daily flights from LAX on Alaska Air-
lines. But be aware that strong winds and storms cause the flights to
be cancelled with some frequency, making it advisable to arrive at
least a day before you begin your walk. Many shuttle services will
drive you from the airport to a hotel in Mammoth Lakes or directly
to a trailhead.

San Francisco Bay Area to the Sierra Nevada The most direct route
from the San Francisco Bay area (SFO or OAK) to Yosemite is to take
Bay Area Rapid Transit (BART) to Richmond, Amtrak from Richmond
to Merced, and a Yosemite Area Regional Transportation System
(YARTS) bus to Yosemite Valley. This combination allows you to travel
from the Bay Area to Yosemite Valley in 6–7 hours. You can also trans-
fer from BART to an Amtrak bus at the San Francisco ferry terminal,
and then to an Amtrak train in Emeryville. It is also possible to take
Amtrak to Reno and the Eastern Sierra Transit (EST) bus south to the
Owens Valley, but this is a longer journey.

Los Angeles to the Sierra Nevada To reach the eastern Sierra from LAX, you must first take the Antelope Express shuttle to Lancaster, and then the EST bus to your choice of Owens Valley destinations, including Lone Pine, Bishop, and Mammoth Lakes. Bus connections allow you make the journey from Los Angeles to Mammoth Lakes, or vice versa, in a long day. YARTS then provides a daily bus service between Mammoth Lakes and Yosemite Valley. Unfortunately, the bus connections do not currently allow you to reach Yosemite Valley the same day you leave Bishop or Lone Pine, as all Yosemite-bound services depart from Mammoth Lakes in the morning. Instead, you must spend a night in Mammoth Lakes before continuing your journey north. An alternative is to fly from LAX to the small airport in Merced, and then continue with YARTS to Yosemite Valley, a faster way to begin your journey.

You will use these same transport options to return to an airport at the end of your hike. If you finish at Whitney Portal and need to reach San Francisco, you will take the afternoon bus from Lone Pine to Mammoth Lakes and in the morning take the YARTS bus back to Yosemite Valley and retrace your route to San Francisco. Alternatively you can take an EST bus south from Lone Pine toward Los Angeles. From Yosemite Valley YARTS buses can take you to the Merced airport or Amtrak station or across to Mammoth Lakes.

Shuttling Yourself to the Correct Trailhead

Those driving to the Sierra face the complicated task of getting back to their vehicles at the end of their walks—this is not trivial, as the drive from Whitney Portal to Yosemite Valley is 4 hours. Options include using a shuttle service (see page 17) or shuttling your own car(s) and using the public transit routes between Yosemite Valley and Lone Pine described on page 16. Regardless of the method you select, it is best to position your car at your endpoint before beginning your walk—it is very difficult to predict weeks in advance an exact time to meet a person or a bus, whereas you have more control over your schedule before beginning your walk. There is no pre-organized shuttle service to Whitney Portal, but if you are willing to hitchhike to Lone Pine (or pay for a private shuttle), you can then use the EST bus to reach Mammoth Lakes in the late afternoon, spend a night in Mammoth Lakes, and continue to Yosemite Valley in the morning with YARTS. Two related options are to rent a car in Mammoth Lakes for a day and use it to shuttle your own car to Whitney Portal or to hire a service to shuttle you just from Whitney Portal to Mammoth Lakes; in either case, you would continue on to Yosemite Valley with YARTS.

The table below lists the route and frequency of each of the transit services; because they are subject to change, make sure to check the schedules and fares on the agencies' websites. Although not listed below, there are also a collection of different shuttle buses in the Mammoth Lakes Basin, including a mandatory shuttle between Mammoth Mountain and Reds Meadow/Devils Postpile that runs 7 a.m.–7 p.m. daily in summer.

Transit Agency Contact Information

AGENCY	TYPE	WEBSITE	PHONE
Amtrak	Train and bus	amtrak.com	800-AMTRAK-2 (800-268-7222)
Antelope Valley Airport Express	Bus	antelopeexpress.com	800-251-2529
BART (Bay Area Rapid Transit)	Commuter Rail	bart.gov	510-465-2278
Eastern Sierra Transit (EST)	Bus	estransit.com/CMS	760-872-1901 or 800-922-1930
YARTS (Yosemite Area Regional Transit System)	Bus	yarts.com	877-989-2787

Transit Route Information

ROUTE	AGENCY	HOURS	FREQUENCY
SFO or OAK ←→ Richmond	BART	1	Every 20–30 minutes
SFO ←→ Embarcadero (SF Financial Center)	BART	0.5	Every 20–30 minutes
SF Financial Center ←→ Emeryville	Amtrak (bus)	0.5	Timed to meet each train to/from Merced or Reno
Richmond or Emeryville ←→ Merced	Amtrak	2.5	4 times daily
Richmond or Emeryville ←→ Reno	Amtrak (train + bus)	6	3–4 times daily
Merced Amtrak station ←→ Yosemite Valley	YARTS	3	5–6 times daily
Mammoth Lakes ←→ Tuolumne Meadows ←→ Yosemite Valley	YARTS	4	Once daily, in the morning (July, Aug.); Sat.–Sun. only (June, Sept.)
Mammoth Lakes ←→ Tuolumne Meadows	YARTS	2	3 times daily, all in the morning (July, Aug.); Sat.–Sun. only (June, Sept.)
Bishop ←→ Lone Pine	EST	1	2–3 times a day, Mon.–Fri.; no Sat.–Sun. service
Bishop ←→ Mammoth Lakes	EST	1	3 times a day, Mon.–Fri.; no Sat.–Sun. service
Lone Pine ←→ Mammoth Lakes ←→ Reno	EST	5	Once a day, Mon., Tues., Thurs., Fri.
Mammoth Lakes ←→ Lancaster	EST	6	Once a day, Mon., Wed., Fri.
Lancaster ←→ LAX	Antelope Express	2	7 times daily

Rental Car Choices

All major car rental companies operate out of the three large airports described above: LAX, SFO, and OAK. Unfortunately, none usually offer one-way car rentals to Mammoth Lakes; if you can convince them otherwise, this would be an alternative to using public transit to reach the Sierra at the beginning of your trip. Mammoth Lakes and Bishop do, however, have two rental car companies, should you choose to rent an extra car for a day to complete your own car shuttle:

> **Mammoth Car Rentals (Hertz independent licensee)**
> 3218 Main St., Mammoth Lakes, CA 93546 (inside Kittredge Sports)
> 760-934-7004
>
> 1200 Airport Rd., Mammoth Lakes, CA 93546
> 760-934-2271
>
> 107 S Main St., Bishop, CA 93514
> 760-872-2272
> **mammothcarrentals.com; hertz.com**
> *Hertz may sometimes allow drop-offs at a different location from pickup.*
>
> **Enterprise**
> 85 Airport Rd., Mammoth Lakes, CA 93546
> 760-924-1094
> 187 W Line St., Bishop, CA 93514
> 760-873-3704; **enterprise.com**

Charter Services

In addition to scheduled transportation, the businesses and people listed below provide private shuttles between trailheads. If you are completing a car shuttle for a section hike, rates will be lower if you select a shuttle service based closer to the locations you are shuttling between.

> **East Side Sierra Shuttle (Paul Fretheim)**
> 760-878-8047 or 760-878-9155
> **eastsidesierrashuttle.com** (based in Independence)
>
> **Mt. Whitney Shuttle Service**
> 760-876-1915
> **mountwhitneyshuttle.com** (based in Lone Pine)
>
> **Mammoth Taxi**
> 760-937-8294; **mammoth-taxi.com**
>
> **Dave Sheldon**
> 760-876-8232 (based in Lone Pine)

Eastern Sierra Transit Dial-a-Ride
760-873-7173; **estransit.com/CMS**
Door-to-door van service within the communities of Mammoth Lakes, Bishop, and Lone Pine

Additional information is available at the following websites:
climber.org/data/shuttles.html
groups.yahoo.com/neo/groups/johnmuirtrail/info
whitneyportalstore.com (search message board archives)

Trailhead Logistics

Before you begin (or end) your hike along the JMT, you will need to reach your beginning trailhead and get a good night's sleep. Below is a brief description of the JMT's endpoints, Yosemite Valley and Whitney Portal, as well as Tuolumne Meadows, and what camping options exist at each location.

Yosemite Valley

Any amenities you need exist toward the eastern end of Yosemite Valley, either around Yosemite Village or Curry Village. Of particular interest to JMT hikers is the large store in Yosemite Village. The wilderness permit office and a visitor center are just northwest of the store. Yosemite Village and Curry Village also have a number of restaurants. Once you are in Yosemite Valley, it is best to park your car and use the free shuttle bus to get around, as parking is difficult.

For your time in Yosemite Valley, you can either reserve a drive-to campsite in one of the valley's several campgrounds (through **reserve usa.com**) or use the dedicated backpacker's campground. Reservations are neither required nor available for the latter, but you may only stay here the day before or after your trip (or two days if arriving by bus); your wilderness permit is required as evidence, and it costs $5 per person per night. The backpacker's campground is located at the back of North Pines Campground; once near sites 331–335, cross Tenaya Creek on a footbridge. Although you can drive a car to within a few minutes' walk of this campsite to unload, you must park your car in the nearby backpacker's parking lot for the night. If you wish to reserve a standard campground, it is recommended that you do so within 10 seconds of them becoming available, at 7 a.m. on the 15th of the month, four months in advance.

The Yosemite Valley wilderness office, Muir Trail Ranch, and the Whitney Portal Trailhead have scales if you wish to weigh your pack.

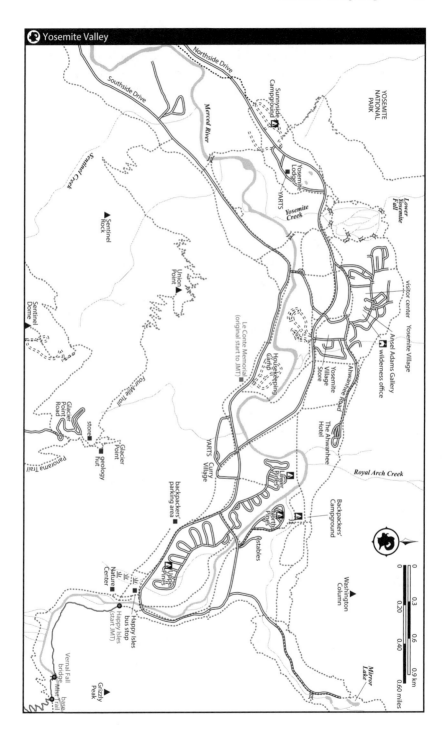

Tuolumne Meadows

Accessed by CA 120, Tuolumne Meadows lies in eastern Yosemite. Supplies are more limited than in Yosemite Valley, but Tuolumne Meadows has a small store, and the Tuolumne Grill serves hamburger-style fare until 5 p.m. Tuolumne Meadows also has a backpacker's campground, with sites costing $5 per person per night. It can be used for a single night by thru-hikers, as well as by hikers the night before or after their trip. Reservations are not available, and you must have your wilderness permit as proof of eligibility. To find it, enter the main campground and head toward the Dana Campfire Circle; the backpacker's campground is due north and clearly marked.

Whitney Portal and Lone Pine

Lone Pine is a small town that lies on US 395, toward the southern end of Owens Valley; by car it is approximately 4 hours north of Los Angeles and 7 hours southeast of San Francisco. Whitney Portal, the trailhead that is the de facto southern terminus of the JMT, lies 13 miles to its west along Whitney Portal Road.

As the base for those hiking Mt. Whitney, as well as JMT hikers, Lone Pine is well-outfitted with hotels, restaurants, and camping equipment stores. The map on page 22 shows the location of a selection of services, including the phone numbers for some hotels. The Mt. Whitney Hostel is run by the same family as the Whitney Portal Store and, in addition to lodging, offers showers for $5. At Whitney Portal you will find a large parking lot, a small café and store, and a campground. The 10 nonreservable, walk-in campsites are $8 per person per night, with a one-night limit. In addition, 30% of the spots in the main campsite are also first come, first served. Unlike the sites in Yosemite National Park, these are not reserved specifically for backpackers, but much of the time you will find a space for the night before or after your hike.

Food Resupplies

Your pack is, of course, made much heavier by the addition of food and water. Most people carry between 1.5 and 2 pounds of food per day. Unless you are completing the trail in 10 (or fewer) days or are hiking only a section of the JMT, you will need to resupply your food along the way—or carry an exceedingly heavy pack. Most hikers arrange to pick

(Continued on page 23)

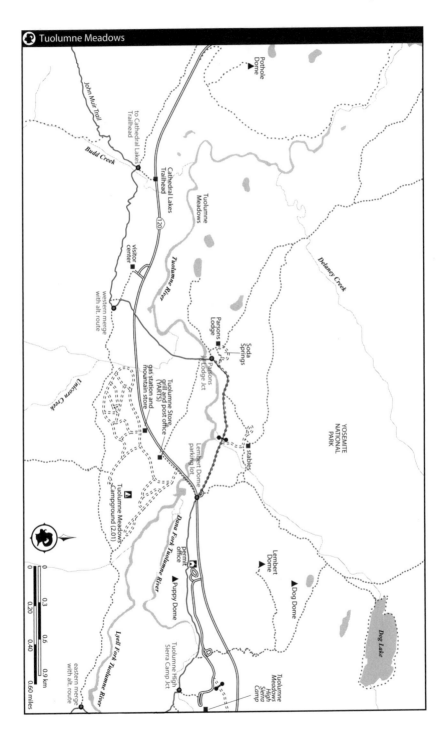

Tuolumne Meadows

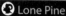
Lone Pine

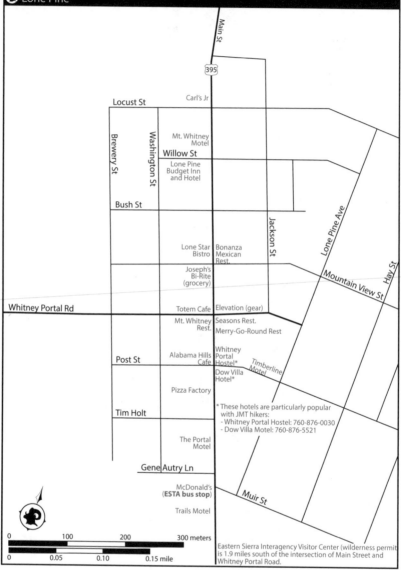

Main St

395

Locust St   Carl's Jr

Mt. Whitney
Motel
Willow St
Lone Pine
Budget Inn
and Hotel

Brewery St

Washington St

Bush St

Jackson St

Lone Pine Ave

Lone Star   Bonanza
Bistro   Mexican
              Rest.
Joseph's
Bi-Rite
(grocery)

Whitney Portal Rd   Totem Cafe   Elevation (gear)   Mountain View St   Hay St

                    Mt. Whitney   Seasons Rest.
                         Rest.   Merry-Go-Round Rest.

                                  Whitney
Post St   Alabama Hills   Portal   Timberline
            Cafe   Hostel*   Motel
                                  Dow Villa
                                  Hotel*

            Pizza Factory

Tim Holt   * These hotels are particularly popular
                                    with JMT hikers:
                                    - Whitney Portal Hostel: 760-876-0030
                                    - Dow Villa Motel: 760-876-5521
            The Portal
            Motel

Gene Autry Ln

            McDonald's
            (ESTA bus stop)   Muir St

            Trails Motel

0   100   200   300 meters
|███|░░░|███|░░░|

0   0.05   0.10   0.15 mile

Eastern Sierra Interagency Visitor Center (wilderness permit
is 1.9 miles south of the intersection of Main Street and
Whitney Portal Road.

(Continued from page 20)

up food every 5–10 days. For a few hikers, that may mean a single resupply, usually at Vermilion Valley Resort (the main junction to reach it is 88.0 miles from Yosemite Valley and 132.8 miles from Whitney Portal), Muir Trail Ranch (107.9/111.1), or in Bishop, accessed via Bishop Pass (136.9/83.9). However, most hikers pick up three or four food drops, possibly at Tuolumne Meadows (22.8/198.0), and then at Reds Meadow Resort (or Mammoth Post Office) (59.2/161.5), at either Vermilion Valley Resort (88.0/132.8) or Muir Trail Ranch (107.9/111.1), and in Independence, accessed via Kearsarge Pass (179.4/40.8). Among the choices in the middle of the JMT, Muir Trail Ranch is very well-placed for food resupplies, as it is a short detour from the JMT and is the farthest south of the "easy" resupply options. Faster parties make this their final resupply point and complete the last 111 miles with this food. Others generally obtain an additional food drop via Kearsarge Pass; some have stock bring their food to the Charlotte Lake junction or Woods Creek junction and others hike over Kearsarge Pass. Details on reaching these locations from the JMT are provided in Appendix A.

If you plan to buy food as you go, Yosemite Valley, Tuolumne Meadows, Mammoth Lakes, and Bishop all have shops that sell a variety of backpacking food. The stores at Red's Meadow Resort and Vermilion Valley Resort have a good selection, but smaller stock, and are intended to supplement a food resupply package, not be your only source.

Contact information for the resupply options follows.

Red's Meadow Resort

Accessed from the two Reds Meadow junctions. The resort offers a water tap, showers (for a fee), lodging, camping, a café, and a store (it sells stove fuel). A hiker barrel allows you to donate food or add to your cache. The resort accepts both hand-delivered and mailed resupply packages in boxes.

> **Red's Meadow**
> PO Box 395
> Mammoth Lakes, CA 93546
> 760-934-2345; **redsmeadow.com**

Food Box Costs: $35 for mailed packages. You can only pick up packages between 7 a.m. and 7 p.m. See **redsmeadow.com/pdf/Package PickUp.pdf** for additional regulations and services. You can also hand-deliver your food box; the storage fee is $1 per day.

Vermilion Valley Resort

Accessed from Lake Edison Trail or Ferry, Bear Ridge Trail, and Bear Creek Trail. See the sidebar "Which Way to VVR?" on page 122 for a comparison of these three trail choices. The shortest distance from the JMT, via Lake Edison Trail and Lake Edison Ferry (twice daily, $19 round-trip) is 3.0 miles round-trip. The resort offers a water tap, showers (for a fee), laundry (for a fee), free camping, a café, and a small, thoughtfully stocked store (it sells stove fuel). Cabins are also available; advance reservations are advised. A power strip is available to recharge camera batteries and other electronic devices. You can donate food at the hiker barrel, or use it to add to your cache. The resort accepts mailed resupply packages, preferably by UPS (the post office pickup has limited hours). As a bonus, thru-hikers get their first beer free—and given that there were 37 varieties of beers during my last visit, you have lots of choices and may even drink enough varieties to turn rather pleasant Bear Ridge into impossibly difficult "Beer" Ridge the following day. Board games and a hiker guitar are bonuses for a fun evening.

Contact Information for United Parcel Service:

Vermilion Valley Resort
c/o Rancheria Garage
62311 Huntington Lake Rd.
Lakeshore, CA 93634

Contact Information for United States Postal Service:

Vermilion Valley Resort
PO Box 258
Lakeshore, CA 93634
559-259-4000 (seasonal, at the resort)
edisonlake.com

Food Box Costs: $20 per 25-pound package. See **edisonlake.com /resupply.htm** for additional regulations and services.

Ferry costs are $12 one-way or $19 round-trip. It usually runs twice daily, leaving the VVR landing at 9 a.m. and 4 p.m. and the ferry wharf on the east side of Lake Edison at 9:45 a.m. and 4:45 p.m. The ferry stops running if the lake levels drop too low, and you then have to use one of the trails to access VVR. This usually happens in September, but in dry years can occur as early as late July. Check the VVR website, Facebook page, or Twitter feed for the latest information. For $10 VVR also provides rides to the Bear Creek cutoff and Bear Ridge trailheads.

Muir Trail Ranch

Accessed from the Florence Lake Trail, Muir Trail Ranch is only 0.25 mile from the junction between the two JMT cutoffs. The resort stores mailed food packages and has an excellent collection of leftover food buckets for hikers to rummage through or deposit into. (The buckets are only available to people who are picking up a bucket.) A power strip is available to recharge camera batteries and other electronic devices. The small store carries stove fuel (including all commonly used canisters), batteries, and postcards. The ranch also has a drinking water tap and a scale to weigh your packs. A nice touch is a big shade tent and benches to sit under as you sort your food. Lodging, showers, toilets, and food, however, are reserved for its own guests, including JMT hikers with prior reservations. For others there are places to camp nearby, and Blayney Hot Springs is just across the river (the ford may be very dangerous in early season).

JUNE–SEPTEMBER:	OCTOBER–MAY:
Muir Trail Ranch	Muir Trail Ranch
PO Box 176	PO Box 269
Lakeshore, CA 93634	Ahwahnee, CA 93601
	209-966-3195 (office in Ahwahnee; no phone at resort)
	muirtrailranch.com; resupply@muirtrailranch.com

Food Box Costs: $65 per plastic bucket (additional $2 per pound over 25 pounds). See **muirtrailranch.com/resupply.html** for additional regulations and services.

Post Offices

A post office is located in each of the eastside towns accessible from the JMT. The business hours, street address, and phone numbers for these post offices can be found at **usps.com**. The only post office near a trailhead on the west side of the range is at the General Store at the Mono Hot Springs Resort, accessed most conveniently by the Bear Creek Trail, though the Bear Ridge Trail and Lake Edison Trail also lead in the general direction. Additional information on the Mono Hot Springs Post Office is available by calling 209-325-1710, or by visiting **monohotsprings.com/post.html**.

Remember that most post offices are not open on weekends, so plan your itinerary carefully. The Tuolumne Meadows office is open on Saturday morning but closed Sunday.

Post offices are legally required to hold your packages for only 10 days, so be sure to contact them ahead of time if your package will be there for a longer period of time. Be sure to specify a "hold until" date on the box.

When mailing your package to any of these places, address it to:

[your name]
c/o General Delivery
[name of post office]
[address]
[city], CA [zip code]
HOLD UNTIL [date]

Following is a list of post offices in towns along the JMT, in north-to-south order:

Yosemite National Park Post Office
9017 Village Dr.
Yosemite National Park, CA 95389-9998 (open Saturday morning)

Tuolumne Meadows Post Office
14000 CA 120 E
Yosemite National Park, CA 95389-9906 (open Saturday morning)

Lee Vining Post Office
121 Lee Vining Ave.
Lee Vining, CA 93541-9997

June Lake Post Office
2747 Boulder Dr.
June Lake, CA 93529-9997

Mammoth Lakes Post Office
3330 Main St.
Mammoth Lakes, CA 93546-9997

Bishop Post Office
585 W Line St.
Bishop, CA 93514-9998 (open Saturday morning)

Big Pine Post Office
140 N Main St.
Big Pine, CA 93513-9997

Independence Post Office
101 S Edwards St.
Independence, CA 93526-9997

Lone Pine Post Office
121 E Bush St.
Lone Pine, CA 93545-9997

Mono Hot Springs
72000 CA 168
Mono Hot Springs, CA 93642-9800 (open Saturday)

Courier and Package-Holding Services

A number of individuals and businesses simplify your food resupplies by allowing you to mail your food to them or by picking up your package from the post office. They will then either drive it to the trailhead for you or hold it for you to pick up outside of post office hours.

East Side Sierra Shuttle
Paul Fretheim
760-878-8047
eastsidesierrashuttle.com

Paul will pick up your food resupply from the Independence post office and leave it in one of the Onion Valley Trailhead food-storage boxes for $40.

Mt. Williamson Motel and Base Camp
PO Box 128
515 S Edwards St. (US 395)
Independence, CA 93526
760-878-2121
855-787-4333
mtwilliamsonmotel.com

For guests staying at the Mt. Williamson Motel, the staff will hold your food box, as well as pick you up from and drop you off at the Onion Valley (Kearsarge Pass) Trailhead. For others, the staff will hold a box you mail or deliver to them for $30.

Sequoia Kings Pack Trains (Brian and Danica Berner)
PO Box 209
Independence, CA 93526
800-962-0775 or 760-387-2797 (Danica)
bernerspack@yahoo.com

The Berners will hold your food box at the trailhead pack station for $80.

Parchers Resort
5001 S Lake Rd.
Bishop, CA 93514
760-873-4177
parchersresort.net/backpackerservices.htm

Parchers Resort, located about 1 mile from the South Lake Trailhead (accessed by Bishop Pass), will hold food resupplies you send (via UPS or FedEx) for $25. See the website for additional conditions and services.

It is illegal to stash your food inside wilderness boundaries, so these services cannot leave your food beyond the trailhead. Abuse of this regulation has resulted in the food-storage boxes at Kearsarge Lakes being locked; the boxes were being filled with stashed and sometimes unclaimed food resupplies.

Resupply Using Pack Stock

An alternative resupply option is to have your food carried in by one of the pack stations operating in the eastern Sierra Nevada. Known as a dunnage drop by the packers, this option would simplify your resupply logistics along the southern half of the JMT. Food drops can easily be arranged for Le Conte Canyon (across Bishop Pass), at the Kearsarge Pass junction (or Charlotte Lake itself), or at the Woods Creek junction. Per-day costs are approximately $100 per mule (each mule can carry up to 150 pounds of food) and $210 per packer. Because the mules can carry several people's food, this alternative becomes rapidly cheaper if you join up with some others for a food resupply.

> Find some friends via the online JMT forums, so you can split food resupply costs.

Rainbow Pack Outfitters provides service over Bishop Pass and down to Le Conte Canyon, which is a two-day round-trip for the packer. You can half your costs by meeting the packer atop Bishop Pass.

> Greg and Ruby Allen
> PO Box 1791
> Bishop, CA 93515
> 760-873-8877
> rainbow.zb-net.com

Sequoia Kings Pack Trains (see previous page) provides service over Kearsarge Pass and down to the John Muir Trail at the Charlotte Lake junction. Other pack stations based in the eastern Sierra are listed at **tinyurl.com/sierrapack**.

Cedar Grove Pack Trains provides service from the west side up either Woods Creek or Bubbs Creek (to the Lower Vidette Meadow junction). See below for contact information.

> Tim Loverin
> 559-565-3464

Pets and the JMT

Pets are prohibited within national parks. If you wish to hike with your pet, you are limited to the section of the JMT between Donohue Pass and the Piute Pass junction.

ON THE TRAIL

Well-traveled backpackers will tell you that each geographic area
has its own idiosyncrasies—both natural conditions and govern-
ing body regulations that many people simply haven't thought about
until they arrive at the trailhead. Knowing in advance what to expect on
the trail will make for a smoother trip. The following sections summarize some things you need to keep in mind while backpacking through
the High Sierra.

Where to Camp

There are two pieces to the "Where should I camp?" question—the ecological aspect and your personal preference. From an ecological perspec-
tive, reinforced by the regulations detailed on your wilderness permit,
you should camp 100 feet from the trail or water sources, and never,
never camp on vegetation, including meadows. Yosemite National Park,
Inyo National Forest, and Sierra National Forest always require that you
camp 100 feet from water and the trail. In Kings Canyon and Sequoia
National Parks, it is only recommended that you camp 100 feet from
water/trail, but it's required that you camp at least 25 feet from water/
trail. Within these parks, you will indeed pass many obviously used
campsites that are not a full 100 feet from water/trail; according to the wilderness rangers, unless areas are clearly posted as RESTORATION AREA,
NO CAMPING, these are legal campsites and it is much better to use an
established campsite than to create a new one. The only longer stretches
of trail where previously used campsites are not obvious from the trail
are those above treeline, where campsites tend to be sandy flats among
slabs or at meadow edges. If you choose to camp in such areas, find a
patch of sand that is 100 feet from water and the trail. Please, never camp

on vegetation—it takes years to recover. Note as well that it is unlikely you will find enough sites for a large group once above the trees, because at high elevations, tent sites tend to be small and occur in ones and twos.

After you have taken ecological considerations into account, it's time to think about what sorts of sites you like to camp in. Do you view an alpine landscape as barren and austere or open and free? Does a forest provide you with a sense of protection, is it claustrophobic, or do you simply love looking up at the branches? Is having a beautiful view from your camp or having protection from wind more important? Or maybe you will pick lower-elevation campsites where you can cook dinner faster, where the air is warmer, and where it's legal to build a campfire. If you are traveling in a group, make sure that group members are aware of each other's preferences.

Also, think about the following information to help you decide where to camp each night: you will experience more dew the closer you camp to wet meadows or a bubbling brook; if, however, you find a campsite that is on a bench above the water source or a short distance into the forest, your gear will be much drier in the morning. Likewise, depressions are cold-air sinks, so the edge of a lake or meadow will be colder than an adjacent knob a few feet higher. Mosquitoes can, and (at times) will, be everywhere, but they are most abundant near wet meadows and slow-flowing streams. Higher-elevation campsites, especially those above treeline, might be windy and colder, but they also have more open views, fewer bugs, and better sunsets and sunrises.

The campsite list is intended to be fairly comprehensive at lower elevations, while in alpine areas it includes just those most obvious from the trail. The campsites in alpine areas are more fragile and would be damaged with daily use. However, with just a few minutes of searching, you will find a sandy site for a single tent in most high-elevation basins; I am just leaving more of the searching to you, hoping that each party finds a slightly different spot than the group the previous day.

Evening and morning sun are hard to come by on much of the JMT, as you are usually traversing between two large ridges of north–south-trending mountains that block clear views to the east and the west. Still, sections that trend east–west, such as Evolution Valley, have late afternoon sun, and sections of trail in open bowls above treeline, such as the Marjorie Lake area, will have much more sun than forested areas deeper in the valleys.

There are at least 200 legal established campsites along the JMT, giving you ample opportunity to pick your favorite sort of environment most nights. In Appendix B, many of these campsites are identified and described, helping you select the locations and settings that you will enjoy most. Most of the campsites listed are well-used; because you are one of 50–100 parties that will use some of these campsites in a given summer, this is unavoidable. If you wish to frequent less-impacted campsites, give yourself a bit of time in the evening to explore farther off-trail for sandy patches among slabs or unvegetated forest floor, but never camp on vegetation just to avoid dust.

In addition, you will pass through areas with additional camping restrictions. These are usually noted in the text and clearly signed along the trail.

Food Storage and Bears

In the past, hikers used a variety of methods to keep their food from wild animals including rodents, bears, and birds. These methods have included sleeping with a food bag, hanging a stuff sack of food off a rock face, stuffing a food bag down a deep crack, and counterbalancing food bags in a tall tree. With the exception of a perfect counterbalance in the perfect tree, these methods are ineffective against black bears, which are very smart and adaptable animals. Because black bears now roam all elevations of the Sierra, especially along the JMT corridor, today's wilderness regulations—and wilderness ethics—dictate that JMT hikers must carry a food-storage canister (colloquially, a bear canister). The rangers are pleased to note that there is now more than 95% compliance with the regulations, and few hikers are retreating to trailheads after their food disappears in the night. The bears are meanwhile becoming "wilder" again: sticking to lower elevations and foraging for natural foods. Please keep making the rangers happy.

Even section hikers will most likely need to carry a food-storage canister: in Yosemite, food-storage canisters are required throughout the park. Heading south, food-storage canisters are mandatory in the Rush Creek drainage and much of the Middle Fork of the San Joaquin River drainage north of Tully Hole. Within Kings Canyon National Park, food-storage canisters are required in Dusy Basin and Palisade Basin (off the JMT toward Bishop Pass) and between Pinchot Pass and Forester Pass (and to the Kearsarge Pass trailhead if you are heading out for a resupply). In both Sequoia and Kings Canyon National Parks, food-storage canisters are required anywhere you cannot find a tree in which you can counterbalance your food 12 feet vertically above the ground and 10 feet horizontally from the trunk of the tree. In effect, you must use a food-storage canister in all alpine and subalpine areas, where such large trees simply do not exist. Finally, food-storage

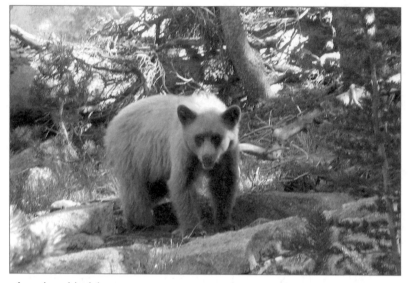

American black bear

canisters are required between Trail Crest and Whitney Portal. Note that these regulations are likely to expand in the future, so check the Sierra Interagency Black Bear Group website, **sierrawildbear.gov**, or the individual parks and forest websites for updates.

Food-storage canister restrictions have now existed in the Sierra for more than a decade, prompting the production of a diversity of bear canisters; seven companies currently produce legal canisters (again see **sierrawildbear.gov**). Of the options listed, the Bearikade is very lightweight, but it is also by far the most expensive and is difficult to come by: it is sold and rented only by the manufacturer: **wild-ideas.net**; 805-693-0550. Many JMT hikers have noted that these canisters can be rented economically. The Garcia canisters can be rented from most wilderness permit offices, and if you rent your canister in Yosemite, you can mail it back instead of delivering it in person.

The need to use food-storage canisters becomes apparent when considering the change in the black bear population in the Sierra over time. Since the early 1980s, black bear populations in California have at least doubled, now numbering around 30,000. Many of those bears live in the Sierra Nevada. In part, this means that even more bears live at high elevations, elevations where enough natural food simply does not exist—and your food bag looks mighty appealing to them!

Stoves, Campfires, and No-Fire Zones

I strongly advocate the use of stoves over campfires in the Sierra Nevada backcountry. Using a stove conserves the finite wood supply that is essential for wildlife and plant habitat and soil replenishment, and it also minimizes the risk of starting a forest fire.

> In all the wilderness areas you pass through, it is illegal to build new campfire rings.

If you must build a campfire, keep it small and only build fires within preexisting campfire rings.

Moreover, many areas along the JMT are closed to wood fires, especially since the maximum fire-elevation has recently been lowered in regions. Overall, campfires are prohibited above 9,600 feet in Yosemite, above 10,000 feet in Ansel Adams Wilderness, above 10,000 feet in John Muir Wilderness, above 10,000 feet in the San Joaquin and Kings Rivers drainages in Kings Canyon National Park, above 10,400 feet in the Kern River drainage in Sequoia National Park, and at all elevations along the Mt. Whitney Trail. In addition, campfires are prohibited at the following specific locations along the JMT: Lower Cathedral Lake (in Yosemite); near the Upper Lyell bridge crossing (in Yosemite); all elevations between Donohue Pass and Shadow Lake; along Duck Creek; at Purple Lake; in the Fish Creek drainage above 9,000 feet (Ansel Adams and John Muir Wilderness Areas); and within 0.25 mile of the Crabtree camping area (Sequoia National Park). As these specifications can change, be sure to study the information you get with your permit on the latest regulations. Also note that in recent summers, fires have been prohibited in many of the Sierra wilderness areas to decrease the likelihood of starting a wildfire—listen closely when you receive your wilderness permit and pay attention to signs along the trail. The summer campfire restrictions may also prohibit the use of alcohol stoves. The campsite list (Appendix B) indicates whether campfires are currently prohibited at each site.

Water Availability

In the Sierra the easiest walking terrain is through the river valleys, not along the ridges. This means that along the JMT water is rarely more than a 5-minute walk from the trail. The exceptions are the upper sections of passes, which rarely contain watercourses, and occasional stretches of trail that traverse a slope. Later in the season side creeks become sparser as they are more likely to dry up, but along the JMT the only rivers marked as permanent that I have seen vanish are the outlet of Trinity Creek (section 4), stretches of Silver Creek above Mott

Lake (section 6), and the waterways around Sandy Meadow (section 12). As well as the major streams, springs tend to be reliable late season and are often indicated on maps.

The abundance of water sources means that unless you wish to camp high (for example, the summit of Mt. Whitney) or dry (to avoid bugs), you never need to carry more than 2 liters (about 2 quarts) of water at a time if you fill up on water before passes and the sections of trail detailed below.

The stretches of trail that are longer than 3 miles without any water or with few options to refill include:

From the headwaters of Sunrise Creek to the Upper Cathedral Lake, the only late-season water is at Sunrise High Sierra Camp (section 1; 5.8 miles).

From Rosalie Lake to Johnston Lake, there will often be no flowing water, but you pass many lakes (section 4; 4.6 miles).

The section from Deer Creek to Duck Creek usually has no water (section 5; 5.2 miles).

The hike across Bear Ridge has long dry stretches (section 6; 5.6 miles).

From the Senger Creek crossing to the Piute Creek crossing it can be dry (section 7; 5.6 miles), but water is available if you detour to Muir Trail Ranch.

From 0.5 mile south of Wallace Creek to the Crabtree camping area, there is no water if the Sandy Meadow area is dry (section 12; 3.7 miles).

From Guitar Lake (or 0.8 miles up the trail) to Trail Camp (east of Mt. Whitney) there is no water (sections 12 and 13; 9.2 miles).

Water Purification, Water Quality, and Camp Hygiene

There is ongoing debate as to whether most water in the Sierra is safe to drink untreated, but there is a clear consensus that backpackers have a responsibility not to pollute waterways. For the last several decades, hikers in the Sierra Nevada have been advised to filter all their water because of potential contamination from the protozoan *Giardia lamblia*, which causes diarrhea and abdominal pain. (Note that symptoms begin one to three weeks following exposure.) As a result, most hikers now use a filter, ultraviolet light purifier, or iodine or chlorine tablets or solution to purify their water. This recommendation remains the status quo, and I certainly do not contest it.

The source and extent of giardia contamination was long unknown. Over the past 15 years, studies by University of California, Davis, researchers Robert Derlet, Robert Rockwell, and colleagues indicate not only that the prevalence of giardia in Sierra waters has been far overstated, but also that a number of other, and potentially nastier, microbes have been detected in Sierra waters. Interestingly, their recent research suggests that the prevalence of algal mats is a good proxy for the likelihood of water contamination. Sierran waters are naturally nutrient-poor, limiting the growth of algal mats that provide an ideal habitat for the bacterium *E. coli* and other coliform bacteria, as well as giardia and a second protozoan, cryptosporidium. In the Sierra, the primary source of excess nutrients in water is from the manure from domestic animals, especially cattle. (*Note:* Cattle grazing does not occur along the JMT corridor, although it affects large areas in the Sierra to the south, north, east, and west.) Areas with high stock use show the next greatest increase in algal mats, followed by areas frequented mostly by hikers, while waters in little-visited areas have the lowest prevalence of algal mats. These results correspond with data they have collected on the concentrations of disease-causing microbes: lakes not subjected to cattle or pack stock, including areas with moderate hiker use, usually contain few to no disease-causing organisms.

Water Purification/Filtration Methods

Different water purification and filtration methods kill different microbes.

• Iodine and chlorine are effective against everything except cryptosporidium.

• UV light (for example, Steripens) kills all microbes.

• Filters do not remove bacteria, such as *E. coli,* or viruses (the latter are very rare at high elevations).

• If boiling water, just bringing it to a boil should be sufficient, even at high elevations.

These studies suggest that many side streams flowing into the JMT are probably safe to drink unfiltered—a decision each hiker must make for himself or herself. If you plan to drink unfiltered water, consult a map each time you stop, to ensure that the creek flows from a little-visited source. And a disclaimer: While I drink much of my Sierra water unpurified, I always carry a method for purifying water and use it if I am unsure about a water source—about 10% of the time.

Despite the fact that most hikers treat their water, as well as the low prevalence of giardia along the JMT corridor, some hikers do contract giardia or another disease-causing microbe while back-packing. It has been suggested that this is often a result of poor camp hygiene, not consumption of contaminated water. Between 4% and 7% of Americans are thought to have giardiasis, most asymptomatically and unknowingly. If you happen to be one of these people, you can easily pass giardia on to your hiking companions through poor camp hygiene—especially since one study of backpackers showed about 30% of people had fecal-hand contamination. This emphasizes the importance of proper waste disposal and food handling. It is essential that all human waste be buried 6–8 inches below the soil surface and at least 100 feet—and preferably 200 feet—from established campsites, trails, and, most important, water. When you pick a "toilet" location, consider not only current water flow, but also that many gullies will carry run-off in spring. All Sierra wilderness areas along the JMT now require that you pack out your toilet paper. A small zip-top bag does the trick, and adding a teaspoon of baking soda before you start minimizes the odor. In addition, if you are a member of a group, make sure that your hands are clean before you handle everyone's food. A small container of hand sanitizer gel is an easy and compact way to keep your hands clean.

In addition, never use soap directly in water. Instead carry water at least 100 feet from a water source and even then use only the smallest possible quantities of biodegradable soap. This is especially important if frogs are nearby. Research suggests that amphibians, which breathe through their skins, are especially sensitive to the chemicals in either insect repellent or sunscreen. Contaminating the water in which they are living can potentially kill them.

Even with campers' best intentions, the Mt. Whitney Zone, extending from Crabtree Meadow to near the Lone Pine Lake junction, simply has too many visitors for the "normal" rules to apply; 5,000 people camped in the Crabtree and Guitar Lake areas in 2012, generating far more waste than the shallow alpine soils can process. As a result, southbound hikers now receive waste bags when they pick up their wilderness permits (even in Yosemite) for use between Guitar Lake

A clear, still alpine lake, devoid of algae, is the best place from which to drink if you aren't purifying your water. The top 6 inches of an alpine lake have been irradiated by the sun to a similar extent as a UV purifier performs.

and Whitney Portal. (If you don't receive one, you can usually pick up waste bags when you pass the trail junction to the Crabtree camping area and ranger station.) Your used "wag bag" can be deposited in specially marked human waste bins at Whitney Portal. Northbound JMT hikers are currently still permitted to bury their waste, as there is no location to drop your filled waste bags once you exit the Whitney Zone. The precise regulations are continuously being reexamined to best protect fragile resources, so please check in at a ranger station to learn the latest policy before you begin your hike. But overall, the system is working! Unlike in the past, neither Guitar Lake nor Trail Camp now has an unwelcoming aroma of human waste.

Backcountry Water

Additional reading on these subjects is available online:

> sierranaturenotes.com/naturenotes/Derlet_Water_SEKI_2007.htm
>
> sierranaturenotes.com/naturenotes/DerletWater.htm
>
> sierranaturenotes.com/naturenotes/DerletSEKI2006.htm

Summer Rangers

A number of summer rangers are stationed along the JMT. In Yosemite there is often a ranger in Little Yosemite Valley and other rangers will frequently be encountered on patrol. In John Muir Wilderness a ranger is sometimes stationed downstream of the Rush Creek junction (near Waugh Lake) and at Sallie Keyes Lakes. In Sequoia and Kings Canyon National Parks (SEKI), rangers are usually stationed at McClure Meadow, Le Conte Canyon, Rae Lakes, Charlotte Lake, and Crabtree Meadows. Some summers, you will also find rangers at the Bench Lake and Tyndall Creek Ranger Stations. The SEKI rangers are typically on duty from mid-June through late September, though budget cuts threaten to shorten their season and decrease their numbers, to the detriment of all hikers in need of assistance.

A few points deserve special mention. First, rangers can be on patrol for several days at a time. If no ranger is present, you may choose to walk to the next ranger station or hike out yourself to report an emergency. Second, remember that rangers have to buy their own food and camping gear, so they, not the government, are the losers if it is taken. They are not meant to be sources of spare fuel and food to make up for our poor planning. They are, however, fountains of knowledge about the areas they patrol if you have any questions.

Ranger Pet Peeves

Wilderness rangers know better than anyone how heavy visitor use damages the fragile natural resources in montane and alpine environments. Rangers stationed in different locations have slightly different concerns, but they all identified the following as the dominant sources of resource damage in their patrol areas: inappropriate disposal of human waste, including toilet paper; burning garbage that doesn't burn completely; illegal campfire rings; creating new campsites, especially on vegetation; and inappropriate food storage.

You can help stay on their good side by making sure that human waste is deposited at least 6 inches below ground, 100 feet from water and trails; packing out your toilet paper; not leaving your full "wag bag" by the side of the Mt. Whitney Trail; not attempting to burn foil-lined garbage, including hot chocolate and instant oatmeal packets; not building new campfire rings; keeping your campfires small; camping in established sites; and using portable food-storage canisters. The rangers do not want to have to start asking to see your TP bags as proof that you have one, but they are getting really tired of picking it up after you. And also of going through fire rings, pulling out all the little bits of foil that didn't burn.

Weather

The southern Sierra Nevada lies between the Central Valley of California and the Great Basin of Nevada. It is primarily influenced by weather from the Pacific Ocean and therefore experiences a Mediterranean climate, with relatively mild, wet winters and warm, dry summers. November–March, Pacific storms bring abundant snow; during these months, only occasional mountaineers on skis access the JMT. During the spring months, the quantity of precipitation tapers, but the High Sierra is still snow-covered. Depending on the intensity of the winter, the JMT country becomes easily accessible to hikers between mid-June, in a drought year, and mid- to late July, in the heavier snow years. The north- and east-facing slopes of the highest passes can retain snowbanks throughout the summer.

Despite the Sierra's well-earned reputation for good weather, you are unlikely to complete the entire JMT without a drop of rain. Make sure to include either a lightweight rain jacket or a high-quality poncho in your gear, with a jacket being advantageous under windy conditions or as an extra warm layer. You can keep your gear dry by lining your backpack with a high-quality garbage bag.

RANGER STATION LOCATIONS IN SEQUOIA AND KINGS CANYON NATIONAL PARKS		
Ranger Station (Distance from HI/WP)	UTM coordinates where you leave JMT (NAD 27)	UTM Coordinates of ranger cabin (NAD 27)
McClure Meadows (Section 7; 119.1/101.7)	11S 345299E 4116961N	11S 345381E 4116952N
How to get there 300 feet northeast of the trail, along the stretch of McClure Meadow with many campsites; easily missed when headed south.		
Le Conte Canyon (Section 8; 136.9/83.9)	11S 358394E 4106306N	11S 358333E 4106273N
How to get there Head 200 feet west on the spur trail at the Dusy Basin/Bishop Pass junction.		
Bench Lake* , ** (Section 9; 158.1/62.7)	11S 372078E 4091162N	11S 372101E 4091371N
How to get there Cross the outlet stream of the first lake south of the Bench Lake and Taboose Pass junctions. Then head northeast, for a total of 0.17 mile from the JMT.		
Rae Lakes (Section 10; 174.4/46.4)	11S 375133E 4074657N	11S 375198E 4074614N
How to get there Located toward the northern end of the middle of the three Rae Lakes. Head 250 feet southeast along the spur trail.		
Charlotte Lake (Section 11; 179.6/41.2)	11S 373686E 4070169N	11S 372820E 4070920N
How to get there From the JMT head 0.83 mile northwest on the trail to Charlotte Lake. The ranger cabin is just east of the trail, toward the northern end of the lake.		
Tyndall Creek* (Section 12; 194.4/26.4)	11S 375972E 4055618N	11S 375632E 4054817N
How to get there Head 0.58 mile southwest on the trail descending Tyndall Creek. The cabin is just west of the trail.		
Crabtree Meadow (Section 12; 202.9/17.9)	11S 379241E 4047246N	11S 379519E 4047234N
How to get there Head south across Crabtree Creek to the Crabtree camping area. Then walk 0.1 mile east along a spur trail to the cabin.		

* These stations are often unmanned due to budgetary limitations.

** The Bench Lake station is a canvas tent that is assembled when the station is staffed. The platform is not visible from the JMT when the cabin is down.

Summer moisture is relatively rare, especially compared with the conditions in mountain ranges such as the Rockies or the European Alps. The summer rainfall the Sierra does receive comes up from the south, from remnants of tropical storms originating in the Gulf of California, the southeast Pacific, and even the Gulf of Mexico. Much of the time, this results in a slow buildup of puffy cumulus clouds, which arrive a bit earlier each afternoon and look a bit more menacing. After a few days comes a day or two of afternoon thunderstorms, before the system disappears again. At times, former tropical cyclones may be entrained in southerly airflow, bringing a larger pulse of moisture to the eastern Sierra. This "monsoon moisture" can result in either a rapid buildup of clouds and/or rain for many hours on end—sometimes even breaking the cardinal rule that "it never rains at night in the Sierra." Any thunderstorm can bring hail to the high passes and peaks at any point in the summer.

Lightning poses the greatest threat to JMT hikers. The clouds can build up very quickly. On many occasions, a cloudless sky in late morning will transform to one with dark rain clouds by midafternoon. Should you see dark thunderclouds gathering overhead, do not proceed across passes. If you suddenly find yourself in a lightning storm, do not take shelter beneath a solo clump of trees, beneath the tallest tree, at the base of a vertical wall, in a cave, or on a saddle; these are locations where you are in greater danger of being hit. Instead, choose a location between scattered trees, boulders, or other undulating topography, where you can squat down and vanish beneath the horizon. Be sure to leave your backpack, which undoubtedly contains some metal, a short distance away. Then, squat on top of an insulated pad or a pile of clothes and get in the lightning position, both to reduce the likelihood of a direct strike and to reduce the seriousness of injury you are likely to sustain if you are struck. The National Outdoor Leadership School recommends squatting or sitting as low as possible and wrapping your arms around your legs. This position minimizes your body's surface area, so there's less of a chance for a ground current to flow through you. Close your eyes, and keep your feet together to prevent the current from flowing in one foot and out the other.

So how does all this translate into the temperatures you are likely to experience on your hike? Daytime temperatures will be pleasantly warm—even hot due to the abundant sunshine. Tuolumne Meadows, at 8,600 feet, has highs in the 70s throughout July and August. At night, you are unlikely to experience subzero temperatures during July and August, but temperatures will begin to drop rapidly come September. But elevation isn't everything: nights are colder in Tuolumne Meadows than at Upper Tyndall Creek, nearly 3,000 feet higher, because the bowl shape of Tuolumne Meadows makes it a cold-air sink. Daily data from the automated weather stations at these two locations (and many others) are available at **cdec.water.ca.gov**.

SIERRA NEVADA HISTORY

In the introduction, I recommended that hikers stop and take in the natural history that abounds in the High Sierra. To aid you in this endeavor, this book is sprinkled liberally with mention of geologic features, plant communities, descriptions of birds that are common in each habitat, and more. In the coming pages are just a few basics on Sierra Nevada natural history. Equally important is an understanding of the people and events that have led to the exploration and preservation of the Sierra. If you wish to learn more about a specific feature or species, many excellent books dedicated to the subject are listed in Appendix E.

Humans and the JMT

Theodore Solomons was, in 1884, the first to have the vision of a high-elevation trail, passable by stock, which followed the spine of the Sierra from Yosemite Valley to Kings Canyon. He was only 14. "The idea of a crest-parallel trail through the High Sierra came to me one day while herding my uncle's cattle in an immense, unfenced alfalfa field near Fresno," he wrote in the *Sierra Club Bulletin* in 1940.

After more than 50 years, Solomons's idea became what we know today as the John Muir Trail, thanks to the efforts of people who explored the Sierra both before and after him. Between Yosemite Valley and Mt. Whitney, features on maps honor John Muir, Josiah Whitney, Theodore Solomons, Joseph Le Conte, Joseph N. Le Conte ("Little Joe"), William Brewer, Clarence King, James Gardiner, Bolton Brown, and Wilbur McClure—to name just a few. Each man helped in the exploration of the High Sierra and the subsequent creation of the John Muir Trail.

Of course, the exploration of the High Sierra began long before the arrival of Europeans. American Indians had used the major passes across the range for centuries, both to trade with tribes on the other side of the mountains and to reach high-elevation summer hunting grounds. Tuolumne Meadows and the northern half of the San Joaquin drainage have the most evidence of American Indian use. Farther south, American Indians did not generally travel along the Sierra but instead crossed over the easiest passes and then dropped to lower elevations.

The first government survey of the High Sierra was during the 1860s. State geologist Josiah Whitney was tasked with making an accurate and complete geological survey of the state. In 1864 he assembled an impressive team of scientists to spend a summer exploring the High Sierra. His staff included William Brewer, a botanist; Charles Hoffman, an engineer and topographer; Clarence King, a geologist; James Gardiner, a surveyor; and Dick Cotter, an assistant. The party was the first to see many of the sections of the Sierra through which the JMT would later pass: the headwaters of the Kern River, Bubbs Creek, and the country along the South Fork of the San Joaquin River. They also discovered that in the southern Sierra there were two parallel crests, the Great Western Divide and the Sierra Crest, and they determined that the Sierra Crest was more than 14,000 feet high.

To survey the landscape, Whitney's team climbed prominent peaks, including Mt. Tyndall and Mt. Brewer. In 1864 King and Cotter made a daredevil crossing of the Great Western and the Kings-Kern Divides. King spent years obsessed with reaching the top of Mt. Whitney, and while he did finally make it up the 14,505-foot peak, he was not the first to summit. Unfortunately, this period of state-sponsored exploration was short-lived: frustrated by the team's focus on exploration and science rather than the discovery of mineral resources, the state discontinued funding in 1865 and later dissolved the survey.

Soon thereafter, Sierra admirers began entering the High Sierra on recreational trips, first exploring the Yosemite high country and then moving southward. John Muir was one of the first people to head deep into the backcountry, ascending peaks and exploring the country, often on solo knapsack trips. However, he was a naturalist at heart, more interested in staring at the plants, animals, and rocks than in producing maps of his travels or scouting routes for future parties.

Among the handful of other people venturing into the rugged country during the 1890s and 1900s, three names stand out: Solomons, who first envisioned the JMT; "Little Joe" Le Conte, son of Joseph Le Conte; and Bolton Brown. Like Solomons, Le Conte was intent on

John Muir

John Muir has become a folk hero as the father of the conservation movement. He was the first president of the Sierra Club, filling that role from its inception in 1893 until his death in 1914, and it is said today that more places in California are named in his honor than for any other person. He is even depicted on the California state quarter. However, his contributions to the Sierra were broader, as he published many scientific articles and was also an energetic hiker and mountaineer.

Born into a strict Scottish family in 1838, Muir's admiration for the natural world began as a child. Disheartened by his early jobs in industry, he came to California at age 30, realizing that he wished to spend his life outdoors studying and simply appreciating nature. Following a brief visit the previous year, he arrived in Yosemite Valley in 1869 and spent his first summer as a sheepherder near Tuolumne Meadows. He was immediately entranced by the landscape, its vegetation, and the geologic history, and disgusted by the damage caused by sheep.

Muir's name became known for his theories on Sierra glaciation: he was the first to propose that many of the Sierra's landforms, including Yosemite Valley, were created by glacial activity. Although he continued his scientific studies and long treks through the Sierra until his death, his focus soon shifted to the conservation of the mountain landscape. His talks, publications, and interactions with endless visitors to the valley established the concept of public lands and conservation in the national conscience. He realized that establishing national parks was the first step to preserving the land, but also that a legislative designation was only the beginning. Next he needed to assemble a group of supporters to help expound the importance of undisturbed wilderness to a wider audience. The Sierra Club, founded in 1892, became his venue. It remains a powerful voice for both preservation of natural areas and the importance of people visiting these locations—for as Muir knew well, the public will only become vested in a national park's worth as a place of national heritage if they experience the wonders for themselves. How fitting that the Sierra's most famous trail and one of its largest wilderness areas are both tributes to him.

finding a route, passable by stock, between Yosemite Valley and Kings Canyon, while Brown simply enjoyed long, exploratory mountaineering excursions.

Eight years after his inspiration to build the trail, Solomons had saved the money and procured the free time to begin scouting this route. During the summers of 1892, 1894, and 1895, he took extensive trips into the High Sierra and mapped a route from Yosemite Valley south to Evolution Basin. However, he was unable to find a stock-passable route across the Goddard Divide. Instead, he climbed through boulder fields and bushwhacked, without stock, through the Ionian Basin and down to the Middle Fork of the Kings River. Little Joe Le Conte accompanied him for part of the 1892 expedition, and in 1896 Le Conte followed a path similar to Solomons's from Yosemite to the Goddard Divide. There, he, too, failed to see today's Muir Pass as a navigable route and instead led his party far to the west and into the North Fork of the Kings River.

In contrast to the northern areas, the headwaters of the Kings River presented a barrier to crest-parallel travel for many years. It remained a challenge to find routes crossing the Kings–San Joaquin Divide, the Kings–Kern Divide, and the divides between the many forks of the Kings. Instead, parties accessed the region by traveling up the river drainages: the route from Cedar Grove to Bullfrog Lake and over Kearsarge Pass, and the route from Cedar Grove over Granite Pass and into the Middle Fork of the Kings River, were both stock-accessible and had already been traveled for many years by sheepherders.

It was by these routes that Bolton Brown entered the Sierra when he made long excursions into the South and Middle Forks of the Kings River (1895 and 1899) and the headwaters of the Kern (1896). Atypical for the period, he was often accompanied by his wife, Lucy, and, in 1899, also by their daughter, Eleanor. For JMT hikers, their most significant explorations included the discovery of Glen Pass (or Blue Flower Pass, as he named it) and the Rae Lakes region. However, he and Lucy were also the first people since the Brewer survey to cross the Kings–Kern Divide, and Brown extensively explored the headwaters of the South Fork Kings River and Woods Creek drainages, climbing peaks wherever he went.

It was Le Conte who finished piecing together most of a route through the headwaters of the King's forks. During the early 1900s, he made numerous trips to scout for possible passes across which trails could be built, focusing his efforts on the Middle and South Forks of the Kings.

In 1907 a U.S. Geological Survey party had succeeded in crossing the Goddard Divide (also known as the Kings–San Joaquin Divide) with stock, via the route that is now Muir Pass. A route across this divide had been the missing link in Le Conte's route, and with this information, in 1908, he set out to travel from Yosemite to Kings Canyon. Excepting a detour up Cataract Creek (south of Palisade Creek), when their horses could not navigate what would come to be known as the Golden Staircase, the Le Conte party's route was very similar to what would become the John Muir Trail as far as Vidette Meadow. Thereafter, he descended Bubbs Creek to Cedar Grove.

As the headwaters of the Kern are less rugged, routes parallel to the Sierra Crest were easily found. Indeed, by 1908 the Kern River drainage was well-mapped, numerous parties had already climbed Mt. Whitney, and a rough use trail formed from Crabtree Meadow to Mt. Whitney's summit.

Ever more people entered the High Sierra with stock during the next years, often as part of the large Sierra Club summer excursions that entered from the west and visited single basins. For despite Le Conte's exploration, travel between the river basins was still difficult; Muir Pass, Mather Pass, and Forester Pass did not exist as navigable routes and most other passes sported only rough use trails.

Only in 1914 did someone on an annual Sierra Club excursion suggest applying to the California legislature for funds to construct a high-mountain trail to facilitate access to the mountains. The following year, limited funds were procured in Sacramento. The legislature gave Wilbur McClure, the state engineer, the task of selecting a route from Yosemite Valley to Mt. Whitney. From Yosemite Valley to Vidette Meadow, the route he selected follows, with remarkable fidelity, the route identified by Solomons and Le Conte. To the south, he initially selected a route through Center Basin, over Junction Pass to the east side of the crest, and back across the drainage divide at Shepherd Pass, as no navigable routes were known across the precipitous Kings–Kern Divide. Only late in the construction of the trail was Forester Pass "discovered" and the decision made to reroute the trail along this more direct route.

Many of the explorers' tales are written as articles in old *Sierra Club Bulletins*, other magazines, or in published journals, gaining them fame for their efforts. Less flashy, less recorded, but equally important are the efforts of the many men who built the trail. By the end of your walk, you will appreciate the effort expended to dynamite cliffs and build switchbacks through the never-ending talus fields encountered over most passes.

Impressively, a rough trail in two sections—from Yosemite to Grouse Meadow (Le Conte Canyon along the Middle Fork of the Kings

River), and from Vidette Meadow (Bubbs Creek) to Mt. Whitney—was constructed within two years of funding. This included completely new stretches of trail over Muir Pass and Junction Pass. However, to bypass the areas that now host Golden Staircase, Mather Pass, and Pinchot Pass, hikers had to detour down the Middle Fork of the Kings to Simpson Meadow and then climb across Granite Pass to Cedar Grove, rejoining the current JMT route at Vidette Meadow. Once good sections of trail existed over Pinchot Pass and Glen Pass, one only had to detour down the Middle Fork of the Kings as far as Cartridge Creek and then climb across Cartridge Pass to reach the South Fork of the Kings below Taboose Pass. Over the next many years, new stretches were built and rough sections were improved as funds became available. The trail to the summit of Mt. Whitney was completed in 1930, Forester Pass was finished in 1931 (only a year after the route was discovered), and the final section, the Golden Staircase, was completed in 1938.

Plants

Plant communities are generally defined by the tree species that dominates a particular community. At the most general level, the entire JMT is either beneath conifer cover or traversing terrain that does not support tree cover. More specifically, the Sierra Nevada's forests can be divided into three zones: the mixed conifer zone, which extends to approximately 6,500 feet and is the only zone where deciduous trees are a significant component; the upper montane zone, which extends from 6,500 feet to 9,000 or 10,000 feet; and the subalpine zone, which extends up to timberline. Above these is the alpine zone, where no trees grow. Only the northernmost 5 miles of the JMT fall within the mixed conifer belt; the remainder of the trail is in the upper montane zone and above, and it is there that we focus our attention.

The upper montane zone spans a wide range of elevations, and the dominant conifer species changes dramatically across this elevation gradient. At the lowest elevations, white firs prevail, but with increasing elevation, red firs and western white pines become ever more common. Western white pines are usually a minor component of a forest dominated by firs, but on slopes you occasionally come across small stands of pure western white pines. At these same elevations, Jeffrey pines are present where the terrain is drier and rockier; usually, they stand alone or in small groups, though larger stands can occur in the lower-elevation river valleys. Western junipers often grow intermingled with Jeffrey pines but are most common on the steeper, rockier slopes, often growing from cracks in slabs. As you move yet higher, western white pines and lodgepole pines intermingle, transitioning to nearly pure lodgepole pine stands at the upper end of this zone. Beyond, you enter the subalpine zone. Whitebark pines dominate these highest elevation stands. The boundary between lodgepole forests and stands of whitebark pines is intricate and usually dictated by topography: lodgepoles dominate in flats and on slopes with deeper soils, while the shallow soils and slabs surrounding high-elevation lakes almost always host whitebark pines. Rarely do you find the two species growing together. In the alpine zone, the growing season is too short and the winter climate too extreme to support the growth of trees. Here you will see only small shrubs, herbs, and grasses, and the higher you climb, the smaller they will become. By the summit of Mt. Whitney even these have vanished, leaving only bare rock and sand.

In addition to elevation, slope aspect and latitude also affect what tree species will grow. For instance, mountain hemlocks are common in the north, often forming nearly mono-specific stands on north-facing slopes from 9,000 to 10,500 feet. However, this species becomes less prominent once across Silver Pass, and disappears south of Mather Pass. In contrast, the foxtail pine first appears south of Pinchot Pass, and by the time you reach Mt. Whitney, it becomes the main species to grow on dry, sandy, or rocky slopes above 9,500 feet. Some general

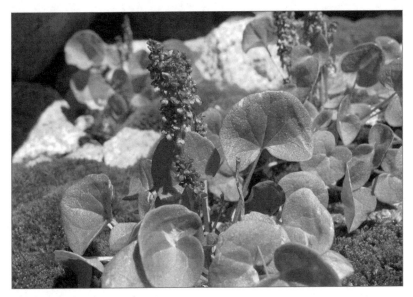

Alpine mountain sorrel

		Needles		Cones			Elevation	
Common Name	Scientific Name	# per cluster	Length	Length	Shape	Bark	Range	Other
White Fir	*Abies concolor*	1	1.25–2.25"	3–5"	Cylindrical, bulky	Bright white on young trees; light gray on mature trees	3,000–8,000'*	Cones never fall to ground intact
Red Fir	*Abies magnificata*	1	0.6–1.25"	5–8"	Cylindrical, bulky	Dull white on young trees; rich red on mature trees	5,000–9,000'	Cones never fall to ground intact
Jeffrey Pine	*Pinus jeffreyi*	3	8–10"	6–10"	Oval; broader at base	Aromatic; thick and deeply grooved	6,000–9,000'	Cone scales' tips turned inward
Western Juniper	*Juniperus occidentalis*	Tight scales		Small blue "berry"			7,000–10,000'	Red and stringy
Western White Pine	*Pinus monticola*	5	2–4"	4–8"	Cylindrical	Patterned, reminds me of puzzle pieces, but not very three-dimensional	7,500–10,500'	Airy appearance
Mountain Hemlock	*Tsuga mertensiana*	1	0.6–0.8"	1.6–3"	Oblong	Red-brown color	8,000–11,000'	More common in north; new branch tips droop downward
Lodgepole Pine	*Pinus contorta*	2	1–3"	<2"	Nearly round	Thin and scaly, not at all three-dimensional	6,500–11,000'	Abundant cones at tree bases
Foxtail Pine	*Pinus balfouriana*	5	0.6–1.5"	2.5–7"	Cylindrical	Rich red color; broken by irregular longitudinal grooves	9,000–11,500'	Only south of Pinchot Pass; long branches of needles look like foxtails or bottle-brushes
Whitebark Pine	*Pinus albicaulis*	5	1.5–2.5"	2–3.5"	Slightly elongated	Quite white and rather smooth	9,500–12,000'	Most common tree in higher elevation lake basins

*Occasionally higher

Note: Other than the first or last 6 miles of your hike, there are nine conifers that you will encounter frequently. They are each easily identified by the number of needles per group, cone size, and elevation range. Here, they are sorted by elevation range.

characteristics to identify each of the conifer species are provided in the table above. The same vegetation zones exist in the eastern Sierra, such as along the Mt. Whitney Trail you follow between Mt. Whitney's summit and Whitney Portal, but because the eastern escarpment of the

Sierra receives less moisture, these forests are drier and more open. Indeed, limber pine, a species characteristic of the Great Basin's desert ranges, only grows in the eastern Sierra.

Of course, in addition to the conifer species, you will walk past at least 500 species of other trees, shrubs, herbs, and grasses on your journey. Most of these species are even pickier than the trees about the slope exposure, moisture availability, soil type, and more: species may prefer wet meadows, dry meadows, seeps, stream banks, the edges of lakes, dry slopes, the base of boulders, cracks in boulders, talus piles, sandy flats, or some other specific habitat. Further constrained by a particular elevation band, translating into specific temperature and precipitation conditions, many species have quite limited distributions. This means you will pass many different habitats in a day—even an hour, at times—and correspondingly many different types of plants. Sporadically through the text, I describe some of the species you pass, a few at a time, allowing you to slowly build up your repertoire. You will learn to identify collections of species that usually occur together and might even soon notice specific habitats and begin hunting for your favorite friends. Should you see all 124 of the species described in the text, you will have identified many of the Sierra Nevada's most common high-elevation species. Look for *Wildflowers of the High Sierra* by Elizabeth Wenk (Wilderness Press), scheduled for publication in early 2015.

Animals

Birds

Well over 100 species of birds have been spotted along the JMT. If you wish to end your hike with such an impressively long list, you are likely a birder, carrying binoculars and a bird book and planning your layover days at the lowest-elevation habitats. Anyone else who keeps their eyes open can expect to see somewhere between 20 and 30 species along the way. In the text, I make note of 34 different bird species that are among the most common in the habitats you pass through. At lower elevations, my descriptions include only the more common species, while the list is more exhaustive at the higher elevations; few species live above 10,000 feet and, as the tree cover thins, they become increasingly conspicuous. For individual descriptions, look at the following pages:

bluebird, mountain: 95	chickadee, mountain: 116
creeper, brown: 75	crossbill, red: 85
dipper, North American: 102	eagle, golden: 185

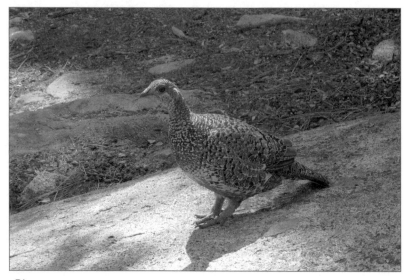

Blue grouse

finch, Cassin's: 85
flicker, northern: 134
grouse, blue: 75
jay, Steller's: 72
kestrel, American: 191
nutcracker, Clark's: 118
nuthatch, red-breasted: 109
ptarmigan, white-tailed: 141
robin, American: 117
solitaire, Townsend's: 135
sparrow, white-crowned: 173
towhee, green-tailed: 134
warbler, yellow-rumped: 105

finch, gray-crowned rosy: 144
goshawk: 103
hummingbird, rufous: 135
junco, dark-eyed: 109
kingfisher, belted: 88
nuthatch, pygmy: 75
pipit, water: 129
raven: 191
sandpiper, spotted: 129
sparrow, fox: 134
swallow, violet-green: 135
warbler, Wilson's: 173
woodpecker, black-backed: 103

Mammals

As most of the many mammal species inhabiting the Sierra Nevada do a good job of staying hidden, you will likely see only a small number of species. You will, however, see most of these over and over again, becoming very familiar with them by the end of your hike.

Most common are the rodents, a group of species that includes mice and squirrels. All rodents' incisors, the sharp teeth at the front of the mouth, continue growing throughout their life, ideal for a lifestyle

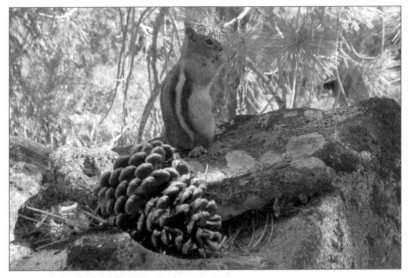

Golden-mantled ground squirrel

dedicated to chewing. One of the most frequently seen rodents is the yellow-bellied marmot, resembling an overgrown groundhog. It lives below treeline but is most often seen at higher elevations, where it is usually seen sunning itself atop a warm, flat boulder. The only common tree squirrel at high elevations is the chickaree (or Douglas squirrel), a small, dark-colored, and very loud tree squirrel that is quite skittish. Three species of ground squirrels make their homes at high elevations. Golden-mantled ground squirrels, which are found from 6,000 feet to above timberline, have a red-brown head and black-and-white stripes down their back; they resemble overgrown chipmunks but lack the chipmunk's diagnostic face stripes. California (or Beechey) ground squirrels, regularly occurring up to 8,000 feet and on occasion up to above 10,000 feet, are grayish-brown, with a light gray patch on the back of their necks and a long, furry trail. Third are Belding's ground squirrels, which occupy dry flats and meadows from 6,000 to 11,500 feet. They are a lighter, brown-beige color and have a short, nearly fur-less tail. Several species of chipmunks occur along the JMT, but they are quite difficult to visually distinguish among, especially because they are tiny and rarely stand still. They include—but are not limited to—the lodgepole chipmunk, which is widespread above 6,000 feet; the largish shadow chipmunk, which occurs in the Yosemite and Mammoth Lakes regions; and the quite small alpine chipmunk, which has yellower sides

Sierra Nevada bighorn sheep

The federally endangered Sierra Nevada bighorn sheep is a distinct subspecies, genetically distinct from desert bighorn sheep that live just across the Owens Valley in the White and Inyo Mountains, and far beyond. Today, the Sierra bighorns live in only a fraction of the range they inhabited when Europeans first visited the Sierra Nevada. The Europeans brought along domestic sheep—and their diseases, which were transmitted to the native sheep, decimating their populations. By the 1970s they persisted in only two limited areas: between Taboose and Kearsarge Passes (now designated as the Mount Baxter and Sawmill Canyon herd units), and around Mt. Williamson, near Shepherd Pass. Thanks first to reintroduction efforts, and more recently to sheep that themselves have migrated into new areas, there are now also populations of sheep on the peaks northeast of Tuolumne Meadows (the Mount Warren herd unit), the peaks southeast of Tuolumne Meadows (the Mount Gibbs herd unit), peaks between Rock Creek and McGee Canyon (Convict Creek herd unit), on the Wheeler Crest (Wheeler Ridge herd unit; this area is far east of the JMT, beyond Mono Creek), on Mt. Langley and nearby peaks just south of Mt. Whitney, and on Olancha Peak yet farther south. Since reaching a low in 1995, the population has been rebounding, and we can hope that their numbers continue to increase in the coming years. After all, as John Muir wrote, they are the "bravest of all the Sierra mountaineers," and they exist only in these mountains.

and occurs only above 9,000 feet. All chipmunks have stripes on their faces and down their backs. Less commonly seen rodents include porcupines, beavers, montane voles (which leave the long soil runways across grassy meadows), and several types of mice.

There are also two species in the rabbit family that you might encounter. The white-tailed jackrabbit is large and inhabits subalpine and alpine environments. You are most likely to meet one in open, somewhat grassy basins, such as approaching the north side of Pinchot Pass. They molt from a pale brown in summer to white in winter to match the surroundings. Second are pikas, little round critters with Mickey Mouse ears that live in high-elevation talus piles or rock glaciers and emit an

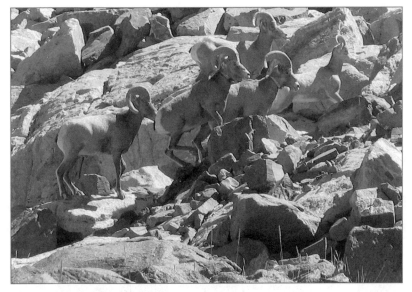

Sierra Nevada bighorn sheep

easy-to-identify "cheep-cheep" when disturbed. Excepting the individu-als living alongside the Mt. Whitney Trail, these are shy little critters. They are also industrious, for unlike most of the rodents, they do not hibernate. To feed themselves in winter, they spend summer harvesting and drying plants and stash their hay piles under rocks for the winter.

As for hoofed mammals, the mule deer is common throughout the Sierra Nevada, except on the highest peaks. So-called timberline bucks even venture well above treeline, while the does usually remain under forest cover. By midsummer many of the does have one or two delicately spotted fawns. While nearly every hiker will catch a glimpse of a mule deer, only a few lucky hikers will get to see the Sierra Nevada bighorn sheep. These sheep require visually open, steep, rocky habitat that provides protection from predators. Amazingly, plants growing in this extreme environment provide sufficient nutrition. Their favor-ite foods include those plants you will see only over the highest passes: alpine gold, skypilot, and mountain sorrel. During summer, the males and females live in separate herds. The females and their lambs tend to live on the higher, safer slopes, while the males are more likely to descend toward lake basins to feed. You may encounter either sex along some southern higher regions of the JMT: both sides of Pinchot Pass and down toward the White Fork crossing, as you hike through the Rae Lakes and over Glen Pass, and possibly just south of Forester

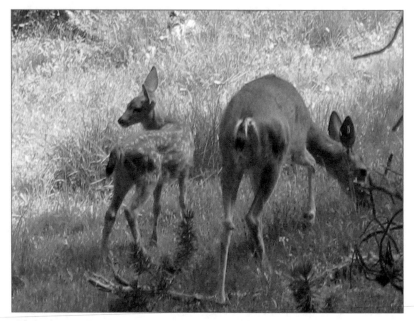

Mule deer

Pass. While there will often be sheep on these slopes, they do a superb job of blending in; I usually see only their little piles of often fresh droppings deposited on talus slopes, taunting me to stare ever harder at the landscape. All I can do is pass on the advice of one bighorn researcher: look for the granite boulders with legs.

The final group of mammals inhabiting the Sierra is the carnivores. Never out of mind due to that canister in your pack is the American black bear, which despite its name, comes in a great variety of colors. They range throughout the Sierra Nevada and, over the years, at increasingly high elevations. Luckily, you need only be concerned about your food, as this species is not aggressive toward humans. Nonetheless, should a bear get hold of your food, don't try to wrestle it away—that food now belongs to the bear. Also be cautious if you come across a mother with cubs. You may also be treated to seeing a coyote, for they are active at dawn, dusk, and occasionally even midday and range into the alpine. Their loud choruses can be both eerie and engaging. And if you are lucky, you may spot a long-tailed weasel, a very skinny creature common across a wide range of elevations and habitats. Between 12 and 22 inches long (including their tail), they are aggressive predators, seeking out just about any rodent or bird. I once watched one (unsuccessfully) try to raid a marmot's den, and I discovered that a mother marmot can actually run very fast and be quite aggressive. Many other carnivores inhabit the High Sierra but are rarely seen. They include mountain lions, bobcats, martens, short-tailed weasels, and, at slightly lower elevations, raccoons, skunks, and fishers.

Reptiles, Amphibians, and Fish

Only a few snakes and lizards inhabit the high elevations of the Sierra Nevada. The most common snake at high elevations is the western terrestrial garter snake, which can occur in wet areas up to 12,000 feet. Long and skinny, with a bright yellow line running down the center of their black backs, they are most commonly seen in marshy grasslands, moving rapidly through the grasses or swimming elegantly in shallow water. (Note that striped racers do not occur above approximately 6,000 feet—all the skinny, striped snakes at high elevations are garter snakes.) Western rattlesnakes, which are venomous, can occur as high as 10,000 feet, but they are much more common at lower elevations. At the lower elevations along the JMT, you will see western fence lizards, with their blue bellies sunning themselves on rocks. Also present are northern alligator lizards, but they tend to hide under plants or rocks and are rarely seen.

Among amphibians, the Mount Lyell salamander inhabits seeps up to at least 12,000 feet, but it is rarely seen. Two species of frogs and two of toads also live in the High Sierra, and the range for each extends toward the 12,000-foot mark: the Pacific tree frog, the Yosemite toad, the western toad, and the mountain yellow-legged frog. Of these, the Pacific tree frog is the most common. This species is just larger than your thumb and sports a characteristic black eye stripe. Its tadpoles are commonly seen in warm, shallow, temporary bodies of water, sometimes in large numbers. The Yosemite toad lives from the Yosemite region south through the Glacier Divide (the ridge separating Humphreys Basin from Evolution Valley), while the western toad is found to the south. Adults of both are usually 2–3 inches in length and have warts covering their skin; the western toad is distinguished by having a pale line down the middle of his back.

In the last decades, the mountain yellow-legged frog has garnered the greatest attention of Sierra Nevada amphibians—see the sidebar on page 56. This large frog, with a mottled brown coloration pattern and light undersides, breeds mostly in high-elevation habitats. A combination of factors has now made them very rare, but you may be lucky and pass one of the lakes along the JMT whose shallow shorelines are still teeming with the 2- to 3-inch-long tadpoles (many different sizes and stages of

A brief history of the mountain yellow-legged frog

Before fish were introduced to the High Sierra, the shallow waters of most deep lakes were black with mountain yellow-legged frog tadpoles, and the banks were thick with adults. The lakes they live in must be deep because the tadpoles take approximately four years to metamorphose into adult frogs and therefore must live in lakes that do not freeze solid in winter. These are the same lakes that were prime targets for the introduction of nonnative trout—and guess what those trout like to eat? Big, fat tadpoles! Following World War II, fish were stocked by airplane and their numbers increased rapidly, while the frog populations plummeted. By the mid-1990s there were (mostly) only frogs in the few lakes that fish hadn't made it to. The fish also changed the composition of invertebrates in the lakes, eliminating many that were important food sources for the frogs. A proposed solution was to remove fish from certain lakes at the headwaters of drainages, reintroduce frogs, and allow both the frogs to survive and recreational fishing to occur.

As this plan was being implemented, a new problem was brewing. In the Sierra Nevada, and much of the rest of the world, amphibians were dying off from a pathogen called amphibian chytrid fungus. The fungus attacks the mouthparts of tadpoles and the skin of adults, and usually kills the frogs as they are metamorphosing into adults, although both young and adult frogs are also susceptible. Many of the remaining frogs in the Sierra have succumbed to this disease over the last 15 years, but small populations of healthy frogs remain. Recently researchers have discovered one possible explanation for the survivors: the presence of a "good" bacteria (think probiotics) protects frogs from the amphibian chytrid fungus. Research is now beginning into the possibility of reintroducing frogs that have been exposed to these bacteria and see if they can survive the onslaught of chytrid.

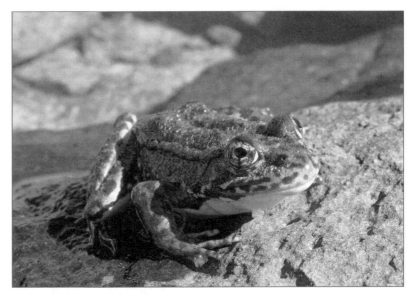

Mountain yellow-legged frog

development can be seen simultaneously)—good locations to search are
the lakes around Island Pass and around Muir Pass. And please note that
amphibians absorb chemicals through their skins, so if you see amphibians in a body of water, be extra careful not to contaminate it with sunscreen, insect repellent, or soap, and do not pick up the frogs.

Fish are native to less than a mile of the JMT: rainbow trout in
the Merced River downstream of Vernal Fall. The steep waterfalls and
cascades along the western and eastern slopes of the Sierra Nevada pre-
vented fish from reaching the higher elevations. Fish stocking began
in the 1870s to create a food source in the otherwise "barren" Sierra
Nevada lakes and rapidly expanded their distribution. As a result
five species of trout are now common throughout the Sierra Nevada's
waters: rainbow trout (native to lower-elevation western Sierra Nevada
rivers), golden trout (native to the southern Sierra Nevada, including the Kern Plateau), Lahontan cutthroat trout (native to some eastern Sierra Nevada drainages and the Rocky Mountains), brown trout
(native to Europe), and brook trout (native to the eastern United States).
Although nonnative, these fish are tasty, and with a fishing rod, a fishing permit, and patience, you can supplement your daily dinners. If the
fish along the JMT corridor are getting too fishing-lure savvy, spend an
afternoon exploring a side basin with fewer visitors.

Geology

It is difficult to even imagine summarizing the geological history of the Sierra Nevada in a few pages—it is, after all, the combination of many geologic processes acting over millions of years that have created the landscape that makes the High Sierra just so spectacular. In the following paragraphs, I summarize the major events and processes that have shaped the Sierra. This is followed by a geologic index, indicating where in the text you will find specific examples of each of the processes described—for what better time to appreciate the grandiose outcomes of geologic events than while walking past them. If this summary is so succinct that it just leaves you asking more questions, as it would me, look at the recommended reading list for several comprehensive titles on Sierra geology. I especially recommend *Geology Underfoot in Yosemite National Park* by Allen Glazner and Greg Stock.

The geologic history of the High Sierra began 600 million years ago when the border of North America was a beach in modern-day Arizona and Utah, while a deeper water environment existed in what is now the High Sierra. Sand was deposited along the beach and in shallow water, while mud sank farther out to sea. As the sediments continued accumulating, the deeper material was compressed into sedimentary rocks, the sand to the sandstones of the southwest, and the mud into siltstone and shale that is now seen in parts of the eastern Sierra (and the White Mountains to the east). This calm period ended around 220 million years ago when the precursor to the Pacific Plate began to collide with the North American Plate and slid (subducted) beneath it. The subducting material was subjected to high temperatures and pressures, causing it and parts of the overlying crust from the North American Plate to melt. The hot, and therefore lower density, magma then moved upward, forcefully displacing the preexisting sedimentary rock. The heat and pressure deformed—metamorphosed—those rocks, creating metasedimentary rocks. Some of the magma solidified underground to become granite and diorite, while a fraction made its way to the surface, leading to volcanic activity.

Each region of magma solidified into a blob of rock termed a pluton. The Sierra's plutons vary in size from a couple of square miles to 10 times that size. In combination the many plutons of the Sierra are termed the Sierra Nevada batholith. Each pluton has a characteristic mineral composition, allowing geologists—and even us—to easily identify their boundaries. We can do so because both the color of the rock and the shape of the individual crystals often change at pluton boundaries. Based on the temperature and chemical composition of the magma, the mineral composition of the resultant granite or diorite varies substantially from pluton to pluton, and often from the edge of the pluton to its center. This is due to the fact that granite is composed of five main minerals: quartz, two types of feldspar (potassium feldspar and plagioclase), biotite, and hornblende. Quartz and plagioclase are white in color, potassium feldspar is a light pink, and biotite and hornblende are black. Minerals like biotite and hornblende, which contain more iron and magnesium, crystallize at higher temperatures than quartz and feldspar; they are therefore the first to form as a pluton cools. This means that the edge of a pluton, which reaches crystallization temperatures first, has more of the darker minerals in comparison to the center. Similarly, the plutons in a region that solidified first have a greater percent of darker minerals than those that cooled later because the chemical composition of the remaining magma chamber changed as the first minerals crystallized.

To return to the Sierra's history, there were two main periods of pluton formation in the Sierra. The first, between 165 and 148 million years ago, formed many of the dark-colored rocks you cross between Mather Pass and Glen Pass, followed by a second window between 103 and 81 million years ago, which formed the lighter-colored granites and granodiorites of the region between Silver Pass and Muir Pass, the Mt. Whitney region, and especially the Yosemite region, where the younger granites are by far the most dominant. The earlier rocks often contain deformed pieces of the overlying sedimentary rocks, presumably because those plutons were the first to push into the older rocks, in the process engulfing bits of the surrounding rock in the cooling magma. These older plutons have much higher percentages of the dark-colored minerals. The later plutons include the lighter-colored granites that are the stereotypical Sierran granites. By 80 million years ago, the granites had all formed, but they were still deep underground and covered by both the sedimentary rocks that formed at the edge of the North American Plate and the thick layers of volcanic rocks that had been erupting overhead. The volcanoes formed an imposing mountain range, probably as tall as today's Sierra, called the Ancestral Sierra Nevada. Remarkably, in the Ancestral Sierra, the major east–west-oriented river valleys already existed in approximately the same locations where they are today; they just drained west from Nevada, for the drainage divide was far to the east of today's.

The following 50 million years, and maybe even longer, were a period where erosion dominated. Subduction halted, ending both the formation of new granite and volcanic activity. Slowly the Ancestral Sierra was eroded away, although how low it ended is unknown. It could have been rolling hills or still an imposing range—this is an active area of research and the jury is out. Most geologists agree that a period of rapid uplift began sometime between 10 to 3 million years ago. There are many lines of evidence, from rates of fault movement to increased rates of erosion, that indicate an abrupt end to the calm. This uplift caused the overlying volcanic and sedimentary rocks to be mostly eroded, exposing the granite. Only in the last decade has the trigger for this uplift been proposed: delamination. This technical term describes the process whereby the bottom of the earth's crust, deep underground, is removed (by an uncertain mechanism). This makes the remaining crust lighter and it pops up. Think about a float in water with lead weights strapped to the bottom; when the straps are cut and the weights drop off, the float rises. While the resultant rapid rise is probably finished (or reaching an end) in the southern Sierra, it may still be staged to accelerate from Yosemite northward, so these mountains are likely to continue growing for millions of years. Although the onset of uplift didn't determine the location of the big river valleys, it certainly deepened them through erosion.

More modern events have fine-tuned the landscape. Repeated glaciations, beginning about 2 million years ago, carried away preexisting talus piles from the valley bottoms and fractured rock from the sides of peaks, leaving a smoother, polished landscape. The glaciers also carved deeply into some valleys, deepening and widening them. All the valleys you walk through on the JMT were once filled with ice, but most of the surrounding peaks emerged far above the glaciers; the trimline demarcates the uppermost extent of the glaciers. As the glaciers melted they left behind piles of rock, called moraines. Small glaciers are still present along the JMT, although with warming temperatures they are rapidly transitioning to permanent ice fields, a designation that indicates the ice is no longer moving. A related landform that is common throughout the High Sierra is the rock glacier, a pile of talus with ice at its center; when active they too move slowly down valley. Landforms continue to evolve through other processes as well. Riverine flood events have deposited rounded boulders high beyond the normal riverbanks. Avalanches and debris flows have carved gullies down the steep mountainsides, depositing material in the valleys below. Rockfalls build up piles of talus at the bases of cliffs, sometimes in dramatic events.

Evidence of all these concepts will greet you along the trail:

CUMULATIVE MILEAGE TABLE

LOCATION	N-S	DISTANCE BETWEEN POINTS	S-N
Happy Isles mileage sign	0.0		220.8
		0.7	
Vernal Fall bridge	0.7		220.1
		0.2	
Mist Trail junction	0.9		219.9
		1.0	
Clark Point junction	1.9		218.9
		0.9	
Panorama Trail junction	2.8		218.0
		0.5	
Nevada Fall junction	3.3		217.5
		0.6	
western Little Yosemite Valley junction	3.9		216.9
		0.6	
northeastern Little Yosemite Valley junction	4.5		216.3
		1.4	
Half Dome junction	5.9		214.9
		0.6	
Clouds Rest junction	6.5		214.3
		2.0	
Merced Lake junction	8.5		212.3
		0.1	
Forsyth Trail junction	8.6		212.2
		4.6	
Sunrise Lakes junction	13.2		207.6
		0.8	
Echo Creek junction	14.0		206.8
		2.6	
Cathedral Pass	16.6		204.2
		1.1	
Lower Cathedral Lake junction	17.7		203.1
		0.5	
Mariposa–Tuolumne County Line	18.2		202.6
		2.4	
trail to Cathedral Lakes trailhead	20.6		200.2
		0.8	
western merge with Tuolumne perimeter trail	21.4		199.4
		0.6	
Parsons Lodge junction	22.0		198.8
		0.8	
Lembert Dome parking lot	22.8		198.0
		1.1	
Tuolumne Meadows Lodge junction	23.9		196.9
		0.6	
eastern merge with Tuolumne perimeter trail	24.5		196.3
		0.7	

LOCATION	N-S	DISTANCE BETWEEN POINTS	S-N
Rafferty Creek junction	25.2		195.6
		4.2	
Evelyn Lake junction	29.4		191.4
		2.9	
start of climb from Lyell Canyon (Lyell Forks)	32.3		188.5
		1.2	
Lyell Fork Bridge	33.5		187.3
		0.9	
second Lyell Fork crossing	34.4		186.4
		1.7	
Donohue Pass	36.1		184.7
		2.8	
Marie Lakes junction	38.9		181.9
		1.0	
Rush Creek junction	39.9		180.9
		0.3	
Davis Lakes junction	40.2		180.6
		1.0	
Island Pass	41.2		179.6
		1.8	
Thousand Island Lake junction	43.0		177.8
		2.4	
Garnet Lake junction	45.4		175.4
		2.9	
Lake Ediza junction	48.3		172.5
		0.7	
Shadow Lake junction	49.0		171.8
		1.7	
Rosalie Lake outlet	50.7		170.1
		3.0	
Trinity Lakes outlet crossing	53.7		167.1
		1.7	
Minaret Creek junction (Johnston Meadow)	55.4		165.4
		0.7	
Beck Lakes junction	56.1		164.7
		0.7	
northern Devils Postpile junction	56.8		164.0
		0.7	
southern Devils Postpile junction	57.5		163.3
		1.1	
western Rainbow Falls junction	58.6		162.2
		0.6	
western Reds Meadow junction	59.2		161.6
		0.1	
eastern Reds Meadow junction	59.3		161.5
		2.7	
lower Crater Meadow junction (Mammoth Pass)	62.0		158.8
		0.7	
Upper Crater Meadow junction	62.7		158.1
		1.3	
Madera–Fresno County line	64.0		156.8
		1.0	
Deer Creek	65.0		155.8
		5.5	
Duck Pass junction	70.5		150.3
		2.2	
Purple Lake trail junction	72.7		148.1
		2.0	
Lake Virginia inlet	74.7		146.1
		2.1	
Tully Hole (McGee Pass junction)	76.8		144.0
		1.1	
Cascade Valley (Fish Creek) junction	77.9		142.9
		2.1	
Squaw Lake outlet	80.0		140.8
		0.5	
Goodale Pass junction	80.5		140.3
		1.2	
Silver Pass	81.7		139.1
		3.5	
Mott Lake junction	85.2		135.6
		1.4	
Mono Creek junction	86.6		134.2
		1.4	
Lake Edison (Quail Meadows) junction	88.0		132.8
		4.6	
Bear Ridge junction	92.6		128.2
		2.2	

LOCATION	N-S	DISTANCE BETWEEN POINTS	S-N
Bear Creek junction	94.8		126.0
		2.0	
Hilgard Fork junction	96.8		124.0
		1.2	
Bear Lakes Basin junction	98.0		122.8
		1.1	
Three Island Lake junction	99.1		121.7
		0.2	
Rose Lake junction	99.3		121.5
		1.4	
Marie Lake outlet	100.7		120.1
		1.0	
Selden Pass	101.7		119.1
		1.9	
Sallie Keyes outlet	103.6		117.2
		2.2	
Senger Creek	105.8		115.0
		2.1	
northern Muir Trail Ranch cutoff	107.9		112.9
		1.8	
southern Muir Trail Ranch cutoff	109.7		111.1
		1.8	
Piute Creek junction	111.5		109.3
		3.5	
Goddard Canyon junction	115.0		105.8
		1.6	
Evolution Creek wade	116.6		104.2
		2.5	
McClure Meadow Ranger Station	119.1		101.7
		5.4	
Evolution Lake inlet	124.5		96.3
		2.3	
Wanda Lake outlet	126.8		94.0
		2.3	
Muir Pass	129.1		91.7
		1.2	
Helen Lake outlet	130.3		90.5
		2.7	
Starr Camp	133.0		87.8
		2.1	
Big Pete Meadow creek crossing	135.1		85.7
		1.8	
Bishop Pass junction	136.9		83.9
		3.4	
Middle Fork junction	140.3		80.5
		3.4	
Deer Meadow creek crossing	143.7		77.1
		3.6	
Lower Palisade Lake outlet	147.3		73.5
		3.8	
Mather Pass	151.1		69.7
		3.3	
South Fork Kings crossing at the base of Upper Basin	154.4		66.4
		2.3	
main South Fork Kings crossing	156.7		64.1
		1.1	
Taboose Pass junction	157.8		63.0
		1.0	
crossing below Marjorie Lake	158.8		62.0
		2.2	
Pinchot Pass	161.0		59.8
		3.7	
Sawmill Pass junction	164.7		56.1
		3.7	
Woods Creek junction	168.4		52.4
		4.0	
Baxter Pass junction	172.4		48.4
		2.0	
Rae Lakes Ranger Station junction	174.4		46.4
		1.0	
Sixty Lake Basin junction	175.4		45.4
		1.9	
Glen Pass	177.3		43.5
		2.1	
Kearsarge Pass junction	179.4		41.4
		0.2	
Charlotte Lake junction	179.6		41.2
		0.4	
Bullfrog Lake junction	180.0		40.8
		1.2	

LOCATION	N-S	DISTANCE BETWEEN POINTS	S-N
Bubbs Creek junction (Lower Vidette Meadow)	181.2		39.6
		1.2	
Upper Vidette Meadow food box	182.4		38.4
		2.3	
Center Basin Creek	184.7		36.1
		3.4	
Lake at 12,250 feet	188.1		32.7
		1.2	
Forester Pass	189.3		31.5
		1.0	
highest Tyndall Creek crossing	190.3		30.5
		3.7	
Lake South America junction	194.0		26.8
		0.3	
Shepherd Pass junction	194.3		26.5
		1.7	
Bighorn Plateau	196.0		24.8
		1.9	
Wright Creek	197.9		22.9
		0.8	
High Sierra Trail junction	198.7		22.1
		1.6	
ridge west of Mt. Young	200.3		20.5
		1.8	
PCT junction west of Crabtree Meadows	202.1		18.7
		0.8	
Crabtree Meadows and Crabtree Ranger Station	202.9		17.9
		2.9	
Arctic Lake outlet creek crossing (Guitar Lake)	205.8		15.0
		2.6	
Mt. Whitney Trail junction	208.4		12.4
		2.0	
Mt. Whitney summit	210.4		10.4
		2.1	
Trail Crest	212.5		8.3
		2.2	
Trail Camp	214.7		6.1
		1.9	
Mirror Lake outlet	216.6		4.2
		0.4	
Outpost Camp	217.0		3.8
		0.9	
Lone Pine Lake junction	217.9		2.9
		2.1	
North Fork Lone Pine Creek	220.0		0.8
		0.8	
Whitney Portal	220.8		0.0

North-to-south distances are in miles from Happy Isles, while south-to-north distances are in miles from Whitney Portal.

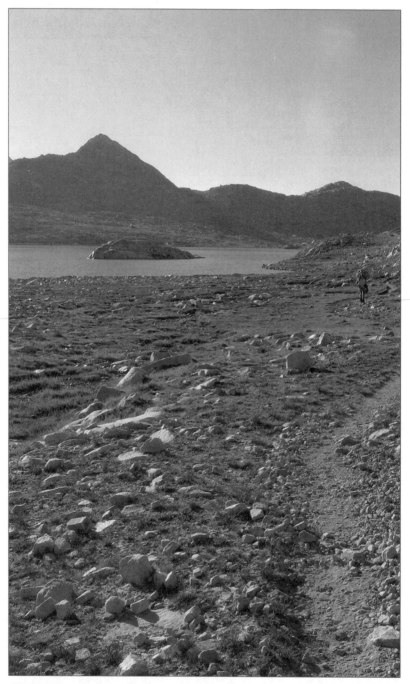

Walking past Wanda Lake in Evolution Basin

NORTH TO SOUTH:
YOSEMITE VALLEY TO WHITNEY PORTAL

SECTION 1.

Happy Isles to Tuolumne–Mariposa County Line: Merced River (16.6 miles)

From the Happy Isles shuttle bus stop, cross the river on the large bridge straight ahead and then turn right (south) to reach the true John Muir Trailhead, a large sign advertising distances to Half Dome, Tuolumne Meadows, and Mt. Whitney. Note that the JMT originally began at Le Conte Memorial, several miles farther west in Yosemite Valley. Today,

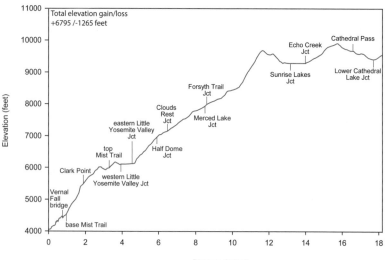

LOCATION	ELEVATION	DISTANCE FROM PREVIOUS POINT	CUMULATIVE DISTANCE	UTM COORDINATES
Happy Isles mileage sign	4,040'	—	0.0	11S 274619E 4178853N
Vernal Fall bridge	4,400'	0.7	0.7	11S 275203E 4178293N
Mist Trail junction	4,530'	0.2	0.9	11S 275439E 4178311N
Clark Point junction	5,490'	1.0	1.9	11S 275776E 4178159N
Panorama Trail junction	6,020'	0.9	2.8	11S 276619E 4177842N
Nevada Fall junction	6,000'	0.5	3.3	11S 277075E 4178261N
western Little Yosemite Valley junction	6,110'	0.6	3.9	11S 277750E 4178733N
northeastern Little Yosemite Valley junction	6,130'	0.6	4.5	11S 278460E 4179141N
Half Dome junction	6,980'	1.4	5.9	11S 278685E 4180304N
Clouds Rest junction	7,160'	0.6	6.5	11S 279499E 4180189N
Merced Lake junction	7,950'	2.0	8.5	11S 281696E 4181478N
Forsyth Trail junction	8,010'	0.1	8.6	11S 281730E 4181595N
Sunrise Lakes junction	9,310'	4.6	13.2	11S 285842E 4185489N
Echo Creek junction	9,310'	0.8	14.0	11S 286129E 4186546N
Cathedral Pass	9,700'	2.6	16.6	11S 287532E 4190048N
Lower Cathedral Lake junction	9,430'	1.1	17.7	11S 287620E 4191522N
Mariposa– Tuolumne County Line	9,570'	0.5	18.2	11S 287789E 4192140N

few—if any—hikers begin with this extra distance, but you could take the shuttle bus to the Le Conte Memorial and then follow the trail that skirts the southern side of Yosemite Valley to reach Happy Isles.

At its start, the asphalt-surfaced trail climbs steeply southward and upward on the east wall of the river canyon. You'll have plenty of company from here to the junction with the trail to Half Dome. The route curves around the base of Sierra Point, which was a popular vista point until a rockfall closed the trail many years ago. Continue eastward, high

(Continued on page 72)

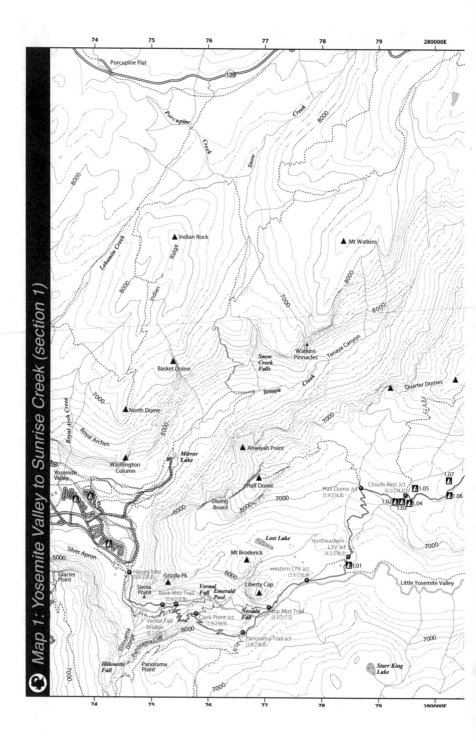

Map 1: Yosemite Valley to Sunrise Creek (section 1)

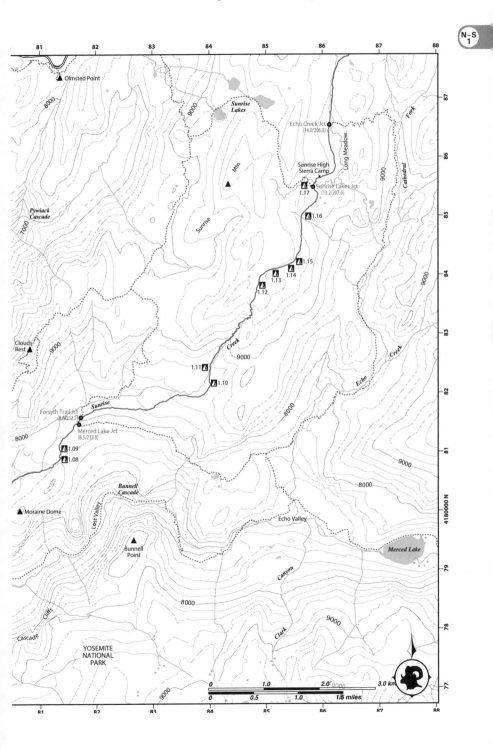

Olmsted Point

8000

9000

Sunrise
Lakes

Echo Creek Jct
(14.0/206.8)

Long Meadow

Fork

Sunrise High
Sierra Camp

Sunrise Lakes Jct
(13.2/207.6)

1.17

1.16

Mtn

Cathedral

Pywiack
Cascade

7000

Sunrise

1.15

1.14

1.13

1.12

Clouds
Rest

9000

Creek

9000

Echo
Creek

1.11

1.10

8000

Forsyth Trail Jct
(8.6/212.7)

Sunrise

Merced Lake Jct
(8.5/212.3)

8000

1.09

1.08

9000

8000

Bunnell
Cascade

Lost Valley

Moraine Dome

Echo Valley

Merced Lake

Bunnell
Point

Canyon

8000

9000

Cliffs

Clark

9000

Cascade

YOSEMITE
NATIONAL
PARK

4180000 N

0   1.0   2.0   3.0 km

0   0.5   1.0   1.5 miles

(Continued from page 69)

above the turbulent Merced River. You descend briefly to cross the river on a stout footbridge [4,400' − 0.7/0.7], which offers a superb view of Vernal Fall; be sure to pull out your camera. Across the bridge are toilets and a drinking fountain that has spouts for both drinking and filling water bottles. This is the last treated water you will find before reaching Sunrise High Sierra Camp. A short distance above the bridge is a junction, where the Mist Trail continues straight ahead and the JMT turns south to begin switchbacking up the canyon's steep south wall [4,530' − 0.2/0.9]. The Mist Trail skirts the southern edge of the river, following stairs up the steep river channel to the top of Vernal Fall. This scenic route is considerably shorter and steeper, and in spring and early summer, it is so wet from spray that you will be drenched once you reach the top. Nonetheless, if you are up for the challenge of hauling your pack up this route, it is well worth the views—and the hot sun will quickly dry your clothes. From the top of Vernal Fall, you could choose to climb up to Clark Point (which has stunning views to Nevada Fall) to rejoin the JMT sooner, or continue ascending the Mist Trail to the top of Nevada Fall. The two trails rejoin at the top of Nevada Fall.

Assuming you continue up the JMT, you will shortly pass a signed horse trail coming in from the west, and then begin ascending switchbacks. The tree species on this slope are unique to this stretch of the JMT and disappear as you climb higher. Douglas fir is the main conifer species, while three broadleaf species are California black oak, identified by its large, lobed leaves; bigleaf maples; and California bay laurels, which have long, skinny, leathery, and highly aromatic leaves. Meanwhile, the ever-squawking Steller's jays (dark blue birds with a black crest) will follow you several thousand feet higher. You will undoubtedly stop and watch these, as the switchbacks seem interminable and are tough on your feet, since many were once paved. The gully you are ascending is the only passable route up the headwall of cliffs. After the climb, you will enjoy a break at the Clark Point junction to take in the view of the waterfalls and the surrounding canyon [5,490' − 0.9/1.9]. Continue upward on the JMT, first on switchbacks and then along a walled-in section of trail that clings to the cliff. By the end of summer, damp sections of this trail are colored by the bright red flowers of California fuchsias and the creamy white, five-petaled flowers called marsh grass of Parnassus. The view from the west end of the walled traverse is spectacular. In the distance is the rounded backside of Half Dome, and to the east, Nevada Fall dropping 594 feet.

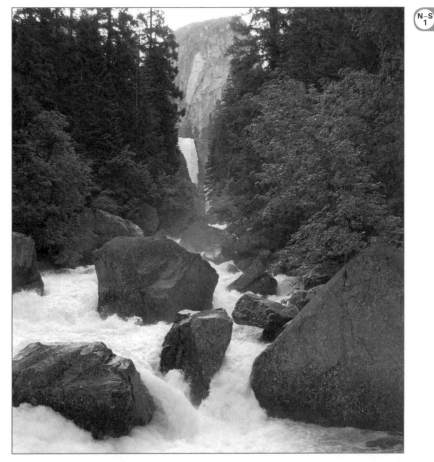

Vernal Fall

Mt. Broderick and Liberty Cap are the two prominent domes across the drainage—in front of Half Dome. While these domes were once glaciated, their rounded tops actually exist due to preexisting fractures in the rock. These fractures cause the surface layers of rock to peel off like the layers of an onion; the technical term for this is exfoliation. At the end of the traverse, you pass a signed junction with the Panorama Trail [6,020' – 1.0/2.8] and almost immediately a second junction.

The trail bends to the northeast, leading to the top of Nevada Fall. A sturdy footbridge leads over the raging waters, after which the trail passes a spur to a fenced vista point, follows a line of rocks across slabs, and zigzags down to meet the upper end of the Mist Trail near some toilets [6,000' – 0.4/3.3]. From here, you climb a short distance up sandy, rocky switchbacks, on which vegetation includes huckleberry oak; Fremont silktassel, with long, dangling tassels of flowers; black oak; and, occasionally, a towering Jeffrey pine, with long needles and large cones. After a short climb, you drop into Little Yosemite Valley, your first flat section of trail, and traipse along the riverbank. In early summer, the western azaleas that line the river are thickly covered in aromatic white flowers. At a junction [6,110' − 0.6/3.9], the JMT takes the right fork, while the left fork serves as a shortcut, and the two merge again a little north of the Little Yosemite Valley camping area. The JMT, mostly under dense forest, roughly parallels the now unseen river, which is separated by a crude log fence. In early season, you may see the peculiar red snowplant that is non-photosynthetic, instead obtaining energy from nearby tree roots. Soon, the JMT turns north (left), diverging from the trail up the Merced River, and reaches the large Little Yosemite Valley camping area, the first legal campsite since Yosemite Valley. Here there are toilets and food-storage boxes. Soon after the toilets, your path re-intersects the shortcut trail [6,130' − 0.6/4.5]. Stay to the right and resume climbing.

In stretches, you climb at a steady grade through a predominately white fir forest, but elsewhere are flat stretches lined with magnificent incense cedars with shaggy red bark and minute scaly leaves. Western rattlesnake plantain, an orchid with white striped leaves, and

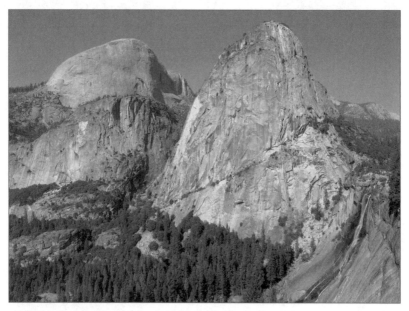

Half Dome, Mt. Broderick, and Liberty Cap

white-veined wintergreen with globular flowers dot the forest floor. A
few sugar pines, with enormous, elongated cones, and Jeffrey pines also
grace the forest. The diminutive pygmy nuthatch, with a straight, chisel-
like bill, and the curved-billed brown creeper live in these forests, the
former circling down, and the latter circling up tree trunks in search of
insects. This is also home to the blue grouse, which is often perched high
in the trees. In early summer, the "whoop-whoop-whoop" of the males,
followed by a sudden flurry of wing beats, is likely to startle you. The
JMT next meets the lateral to Half Dome [6,980' – 1.4/5.9], an incred-
ible 4-mile round trip that shouldn't be missed; just make sure that your
wilderness permit allows you to climb Half Dome's cables (see page 210).
The JMT turns east and traverses to Sunrise Creek on a dry slope with
dense scrub cover: The underlying slabs are close to the surface, and in
many places there is insufficient soil depth for trees. In half a mile, the
JMT meets the trail to Clouds Rest [7,160' – 0.6/6.5], the first of two trails
leading to this worthwhile summit with outstanding views of Yosemite
Valley, Half Dome, and the Yosemite high country (see page 210).

There are a few campsites near the junction, both just before you
reach it and on the ridge to the northwest. Another large camping area
exists just a bit farther along the JMT in a flat forest opening along the
banks of Sunrise Creek. The JMT now follows Sunrise Creek, passing
occasional campsites on either side of the trail. Farther along, a collection of use trails leads north to campsites atop a small knob with
delightful views toward Half Dome and Mt. Starr King, a dome south
of the Merced River canyon. The trail continues to climb through the
white fir forest, with openings sporting Jeffrey pines. As you ascend,
the white firs are slowly replaced by red firs, with much shorter needles and a deep-maroon bark on older trees. The cones of this species
differ as well, but these always decompose before dropping from the
trees and therefore are of little use to hikers for identification. A few
more campsites appear after you diverge from the main Sunrise Creek
and intersect a small tributary. You cross the creek and shortly reach
the junction with a trail to Merced Lake [7,950' – 2.0/8.5], where you
stay left, and immediately thereafter with the Forsyth Trail [8,010' –
0.1/8.6], where the JMT trends right. From this junction, too, you can
detour upward to summit Clouds Rest (see page 210).

For the next mile, the trail diverges from Sunrise Creek, crossing
over open flats as it ascends a shallow ridge. Just steps to your south,
the landscape drops steeply to the Merced River; peer over the lip for a
beautiful view of Mt. Clark. As the trail reenters dry, bare, red fir forest
and then bends north, a few campsites emerge: the first along the banks

of a potentially dry tributary and others where you again cross Sunrise Creek. These are your last campsites for several miles (and potentially your last sources of water until you reach Sunrise High Sierra Camp), as you now begin the climb up Sunrise Mountain. Red firs, western white pines, western junipers, and Jeffrey pines are all present along the ensuing climb. Western white pine has midsize needles in groups of five, arranged on the branch in a way that gives them an airy appearance. Higher still, you enter the first lodgepole pine forest along the JMT. This species will dominate along much of the trail. Lodgepole pines are characterized by small, round cones that are always abundant around tree trunks, needles in clusters of two, and fine-scaled bark. You next cross a shallow, sandy ridge and descend to a meadow, alongside which there are several campsites, although the water source may dry out by late summer. A common shrub throughout this area is alpine prickly currant, with prickly trailing stems, slightly lobed leaves, and edible red berries. Along the entire length of the JMT, this species is abundant from the montane to the alpine regions, often forming thickets along the ground in lodgepole forests. The trail crosses another sandy ridge and descends toward Sunrise High Sierra Camp.

En route, you cross one small tributary where there is a small campsite among mountain hemlock trees. These short-needled conifers with small, elongated cones prefer cooler, north-facing slopes and gradually diminish in abundance to the south. As John Muir described his favorite tree: "The Hemlock Spruce is the most singularly beautiful of all the California coniferæ. So slender is its axis at the top, that it bends over and droops like the stalk of a nodding lily. The branches droop also, and divide into innumerable slender, waving sprays, which are arranged in a varied, eloquent harmony that is wholly indescribable." Be sure to spend one night on your walk beneath their elegant boughs!

A short descent brings you to the L-shaped Long Meadow and the junction with the trail to Sunrise Lakes and Tenaya Lake [9,310' – 4.6/13.2]. Many campsites, food-storage boxes, a water tap, and a pit toilet can be found a short distance up this trail. A spur trail to Sunrise High Sierra Camp is found a short stretch ahead; the camp has supplies only for its guests, who put their names into the reservation lottery months in advance. Be sure to enjoy the spectacular views south to the Clark Range and southeast to Mt. Florence before turning north up Long Meadow, which you skirt on sandy flats along its western edge. Near the Echo Creek Trail junction [9,310' – 0.8/14.0], you briefly enter forest and then reemerge into vast Long Meadow. You now see notably

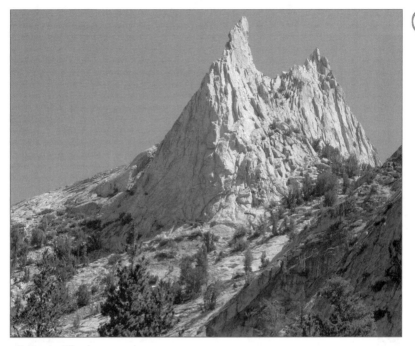

Cathedral Peak

steep Columbia Finger straight ahead. This spire of jointed rock once rose above the surrounding ice fields.

Beyond Long Meadow, you continue the climb toward Cathedral Pass through an open, sandy lodgepole forest. Alongside boulders, you will find mountain pride penstemon, one of the most common species both here and in the subalpine region. It is easily identified by vast blooms of tubular, bright magenta flowers decorating a low-growing shrub with slightly serrate leaves. When you reach a sandy saddle, stop and enjoy the view of the Cathedral Range: the mile-long, knife-edge Matthes Crest to your east, the Echo Peaks and Cathedral Peak to the northeast, and Columbia Finger and Tresidder Peak to the west. For each peak, note that the lower reaches are smooth and steep, having been rolled over by glaciers, while the summits are jagged spires of jointed rock. To enjoy the view from a higher perch, continue the short ascent west to Columbia Finger saddle (see page 211). You now descend the eastern shoulder of Tresidder Peak toward the broad saddle called Cathedral Pass [9,700' – 2.6/16.6] and into the shallow cirque cradling the Upper Cathedral

(Continued on page 80)

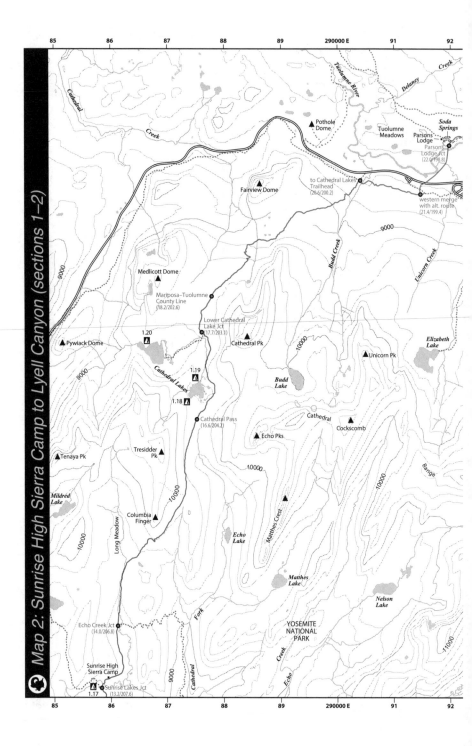

Map 2: Sunrise High Sierra Camp to Lyell Canyon (sections 1–2)

Cathedral Creek

Tuolumne River

Delaney Creek

Pothole Dome

Soda Springs

Tuolumne Meadows

Parsons Lodge

Parsons Lodge Jct (22.0/198.8)

Creek

Fairview Dome

to Cathedral Lakes Trailhead (20.6/200.2)

western merge with alt. route (21.4/199.4)

Budd Creek

9000

Unicorn Creek

Medlicott Dome

Mariposa–Tuolumne County Line (18.2/202.6)

Lower Cathedral Lake Jct (17.7/203.1)

Elizabeth Lake

9000

Pywiack Dome

1.20

Cathedral Pk

Unicorn Pk

10000

Cathedral Lakes

1.19

Budd Lake

1.18

Cathedral Pass (16.6/204.2)

Cathedral

Cockscomb

Echo Pks

9000

Tenaya Pk

Tresidder Pk

10000

Range

Mildred Lake

Columbia Finger

Long Meadow

10000

Matthes Crest

10000

Echo Lake

10000

Matthes Lake

Nelson Lake

11000

Echo Creek Jct (14.0/206.8)

YOSEMITE NATIONAL PARK

Fork

Cathedral

Creek

Echo

Sunrise High Sierra Camp

1.17

Sunrise Lakes Jct (13.2/207.6)

9000

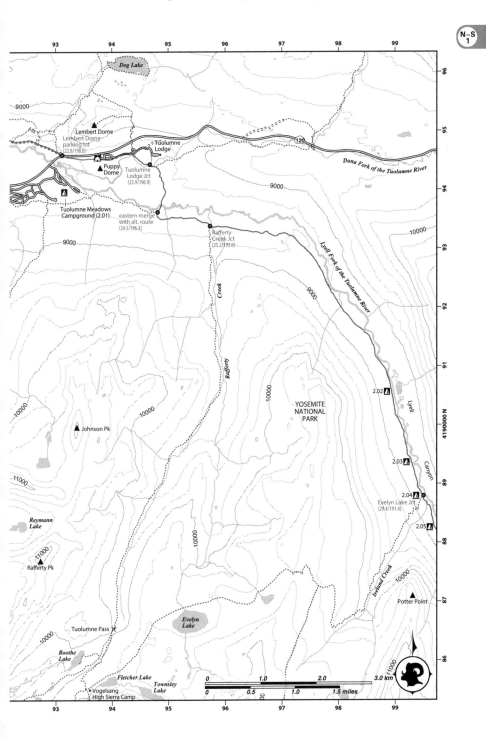

Dog Lake

9000

Lembert Dome

Lembert Dome
parking lot
(22.8/198.0)

Tuolumne
Lodge

120

Puppy
Dome

Tuolumne Lodge Jct
(23.9/196.9)

Dana Fork of the Tuolumne River

9000

Tuolumne Meadows
Campground (2.01)

eastern merge
with alt. route
(24.5/196.3)

Rafferty
Creek Jct
(25.2/195.6)

9000

10000

9000

Lyell Fork of the Tuolumne River

Rafferty Creek

Rafferty

92

91

2.02

Lyell

4190000 N

Johnson Pk

10000

10000

YOSEMITE
NATIONAL
PARK

2.03

Canyon

89

2.04

Evelyn Lake Jct
(29.4/191.4)

10000

10000

2.05

88

Reymann
Lake

11000

Rafferty Pk

10000

Ireland Creek

10000

87

Potter Point

Tuolumne Pass

11000

Evelyn
Lake

Boothe
Lake

Fletcher Lake

Townsley
Lake

86

Vogelsang
High Sierra Camp

0		1.0		2.0		3.0 km
0	0.5		1.0		1.5 miles	

93   94   95   96   97   98   99

(Continued from page 77)

Lake. The lake is nestled in a large meadow and surrounded by the steep lower walls of Tresidder Peak and the Echo Peaks. The trail has recently been rerouted out of the meadow to allow it to regenerate. A handful of campsites can be found on the southwest side of the lake and in trees at the northern end of the lake; just be sure to skirt the wet meadow as you approach them. Note that campfires are prohibited both here and at the Lower Cathedral Lake. You continue descending through mixed lodgepole and hemlock forest. The low-growing dwarf bilberry, a type of blueberry with small, ovate leaves and bell-shaped flowers, dominates the edge of meadows and wet sections of forest floor, but unfortunately, it rarely bares fruit. Continuing, you reach a lateral trail to the Lower Cathedral Lake [9,430' – 1.1/17.7], where you will find additional camp-sites, your last before Tuolumne Meadows. You now make a gradual climb through open lodgepole forest and then onto a sandy shoulder, the whole while traversing below Cathedral Peak. In 1869 John Muir was the first to climb this magnificent peak, via the slabs on the west face, the route at which you are gazing. The trail now leads you to a seemingly unnoteworthy saddle, but this pass is the divide between the Merced and Tuolumne River drainages [9,570' – 0.4/18.2]. There is no marker indicating when you cross the drainage divide, and it is difficult to decide when the grade becomes "downhill," but the results farther downstream couldn't be more dramatic: Water flowing into the Cathedral Lakes drains into Tenaya Lake and then down Tenaya Canyon to Yosemite Valley, while water to the north flows down the Tuolumne River to Hetch Hetchy Reservoir and the plumbing of San Francisco. This hasn't always been the case, however, for glaciers once filled Tuolumne Meadow to the top of this pass, such that there were two outflows from Tuolumne Meadows, one down the Tuolumne River canyon and a second into Tenaya Lake.

SECTION 2.

Tuolumne–Mariposa County Line to Donohue Pass: Tuolumne River (17.9 miles)

Slowly, the slope increases, crossing sandy flats before dropping more steeply past a robust spring and then crossing the small stream flowing from it. You descend on switchbacks through a forest dominated by mountain hemlock mixed with occasional western white pines. Where the grade lessens, you cross Cathedral Creek on rock and then traverse an avalanche zone with stunted trees; Fairview Dome dominates the view to the northwest. A second descent through a drier forest—this one dominated by lodgepole pines—brings you to a junction, just south of CA 120, where a large map of the area is posted [8,600' – 2.5/20.6]. Continuing straight ahead 0.1 mile would bring you to the Cathedral Lakes parking area and a (free) Tuolumne Meadows shuttle bus stop, while the JMT continues east on a trail that roughly

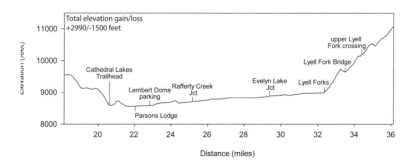

LOCATION	ELEVATION	DISTANCE FROM PREVIOUS POINT	CUMULATIVE DISTANCE	UTM COORDINATES
Mariposa–Tuolumne County Line	9,570'	—	18.2	11S 287789E 4192140N
trail to Cathedral Lakes Trailhead	8,600'	2.4	20.6	11S 290409E 4194106N
western merge with Tuolumne perimeter trail	8,630'	0.8	21.4	11S 291480E 4193871N
Parsons Lodge junction	8,560'	0.6	22.0	11S 291982E 4194705N
Lembert Dome parking lot	8,590'	0.8	22.8	11S 293123E 4194590N
Tuolumne Meadows Lodge junction	8,680'	1.1	23.9	11S 294682E 4194429N
eastern merge with Tuolumne perimeter trail	8,670'	0.6	24.5	11S 294819E 4193619N
Rafferty Creek junction	8,720'	0.7	25.2	11S 295742E 4193386N
Evelyn Lake junction	8,900'	4.2	29.4	11S 299493E 4188811N
start of climb from Lyell Canyon (Lyell Forks)	9,020'	2.9	32.3	11S 300899E 4184697N
Lyell Fork Bridge	9,650'	1.2	33.5	11S 300863E 4183358N
second Lyell Fork crossing	10,190'	0.9	34.4	11S 301325E 4182269N
Donohue Pass	11,060'	1.7	36.1	11S 302025E 4181480N

parallels the highway. The trail almost immediately crosses Budd Creek on a footbridge and you climb gently through open lodgepole forest to reach another junction [8,630' – 0.8/21.4]. At this junction, the official JMT (and therefore the route described here) heads north through Tuolumne Meadows and past the historic Parsons Lodge. While many hikers opt to continue east on the trail paralleling CA 120, a more direct route to the Tuolumne Meadows campground, I encourage you to walk out into Tuolumne Meadows, either with your pack or later for an evening excursion. If you choose the shorter route, head due east, ignoring all junctions: past the Elizabeth Lake junction (turning north here leads you into the campground and the most direct route to the store), past the campground, continuing for approximately 2.3 miles through an open lodgepole forest until you rejoin the JMT just after it has crossed the bridge across the Lyell Fork of the Tuolumne.

Before you continue, a little Tuolumne Meadows orientation: Tuolumne Meadows amenities exist along the 1.5-mile east–west CA 120 corridor beginning where the two possible routes diverge. From west to east, you will encounter a visitor center with an excellent bookstore and natural history displays, a small mountaineering store, the Tuolumne Meadows Grill, the grocery store, and the campground, the only legal camping you'll find between the Lower Cathedral Lake and the "4-mile mark" up Lyell Canyon. The Tuolumne Meadows campground has a section of walk-in campgrounds reserved for backpackers: These are due south of the Dana Campfire Circle and toward the eastern end of the campground, cost $5 per person, and allow only a one-night stay. (See page 21 for a detailed map of Tuolumne Meadows.) Farther east, along a spur road, is first the wilderness permit station, and then, after a mile, the Tuolumne Meadows Lodge, where meals and lodging are available, but must be reserved well in advance.

To follow the official, and certainly more scenic, JMT route, turn north (left) at the previously described junction. Just around the corner, the trail passes a junction to the visitor center and then reaches CA 120. Cross the road and enter wide-open, flower-filled Tuolumne Meadows, following the metal sign to Parsons Lodge. As the trail cuts north across the meadows, stop frequently and stare in all directions, enjoying the landscape of nearby domes, Unicorn and Cathedral Peaks, and the large, red, rounded peaks to the east, Mt. Dana and Mt. Gibbs. Pothole Dome, to the west, and Lembert Dome, to the east, are good examples of roches moutonnées. These formed as a glacier flowed up and over their tops. The ascending side is smooth and gentle, while the glacier plucked large chunks of rock on the downhill side, creating a jagged, steep topography. You may also note the young lodgepole pines encroaching on the meadows. Researchers have several hypotheses for their relentless invasion but have not yet reached a consensus on the cause. You cross the Tuolumne River on a footbridge below some buildings, Parsons Lodge and McCauley Cabin, at which you should stop and take a look [8,560' – 0.7/22.0]. The Sierra Club built Parsons Lodge in 1915 as a mountain meeting room, and it is filled with written and photographic tales of historical Tuolumne. From Parsons Lodge, your path heads past the Soda Springs, where early tourists came to sample the soda water and relax. This was one of John Muir's favorite hangouts in Tuolumne, and where he conceived the idea of establishing Yosemite National Park. When you are ready to continue, the ever-present carved metal trail signs keep you headed eastward through the meadow, now on the route of the original CA 120.

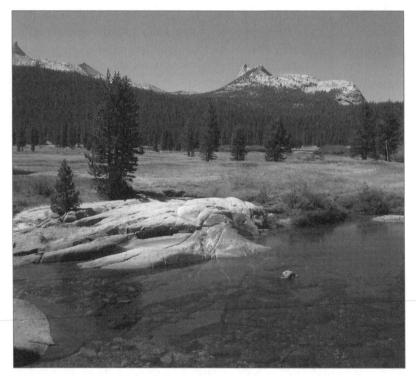

Tuolumne Meadows with Cathedral Peak in the background

As you head east toward the steep granite face of Lembert Dome, take some time to read the informative signs along the road, describing both the human and natural history of the area. Approaching the dome, you circumvent a gate that bars vehicular traffic and pass a spur road to the local stables. Keeping to the road, you pass below the dome and through its parking lot to reach the highway [8,590' – 0.8/22.8]. The summit of Lembert Dome provides a 360-degree vista of the Tuolumne Meadows area; if you have a few hours, consider climbing to its summit (see page 211). Cross the highway again, and pick up a wide dirt track to a large parking lot and the wilderness permit station, where rangers can both dispense wilderness permits and answer questions you pose regarding conditions. But please note that they are permitted only to dispense the most recent factual information available to them, and not to offer advice. Your route now parallels the road to the Tuolumne Meadows Lodge. You pass another large backpacker's parking lot (and the most direct route to Lembert Dome) and then curve southeast toward the Dana Fork of the Tuolumne River. Pass a signed spur trail to the Tuolumne Meadows Lodge (also known as the Tuolumne Meadows High Sierra Camp) [8,680' – 1.0/23.9]; turn right to cross the Dana Fork on a footbridge, and quickly reach a junction with a trail headed northeast along the Dana Fork, continuing eventually to Gaylor Lakes. Staying on the JMT, you curve south (right) and leave the Dana Fork drainage. Without realizing it, you've just climbed across a drainage divide, and the trail suddenly exits the dry lodgepole forest and reaches the Lyell Fork of the Tuolumne River. Cross the river on a pair of bridges and look into the water at the exquisitely carved granite—smooth slabs and deep holes, dangerous if the water is high but perfect for a cold dip later in the summer. In a few more steps, you reenter forest and reach the junction where the official JMT reconnects with the route skirting the southern edge of the meadows [8,670' – 0.6/24.5].

As you leave Tuolumne Meadows, you no longer have to worry about heading in the correct direction at the junctions you had been encountering every few minutes and once again can focus on the beautiful scenery. Although you can't see it from the trail, you are paralleling the Lyell Fork eastward, passing alternately through sections of lodgepole forest—which feature little ground cover—as well as through small meadows. Short stretches of slab are mixed in. Although these openings appear grass-covered, many actually are inhabited by a group of related species, sedges, whose flowers manifest in small, dark heads. Sometimes individual plants appear as circles, where they have grown outward over many years. A common species here, and in many other meadows, is Parish's yampah, a member of the carrot family that has three linear leaf-lobes and a broad head of minute white flowers. Two species of pussytoes are also abundant at the meadow edges. These species form extensive mats, have small, elongated, and quite fuzzy leaves, and feature flowers that resemble tiny tufts of fuzz. Rosy pussytoes' flowers have a pinkish tinge, while others, such as meadow pussytoes, are white. The meadows are a favorite haunt of mule deer. The bucks that dwell in the sanctuary provided by the national park boundaries are tame and sport large antlers. Cassin's finches, which feature red heads and streaked pinkish backs, and red crossbills, which are somewhat larger and feature the eponymous crossed beaks, are both present in this forest. Your next junction is with the Rafferty Creek Trail [8,720' – 0.7/25.2], which heads south to Vogelsang High Sierra Camp.

(Continued on page 88)

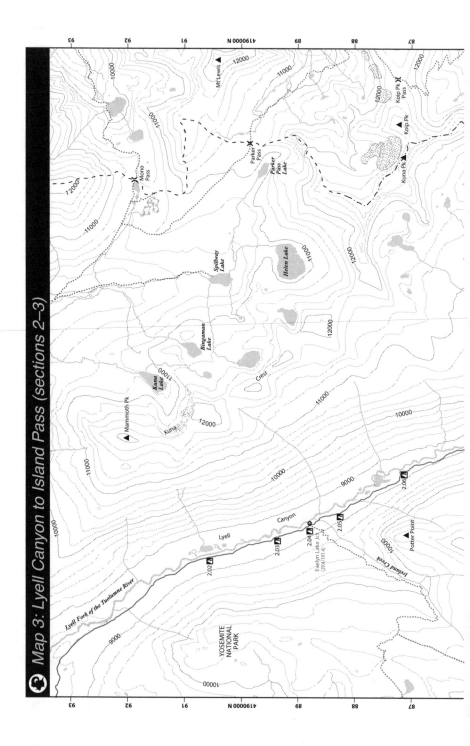

Map 3: Lyell Canyon to Island Pass (sections 2–3)

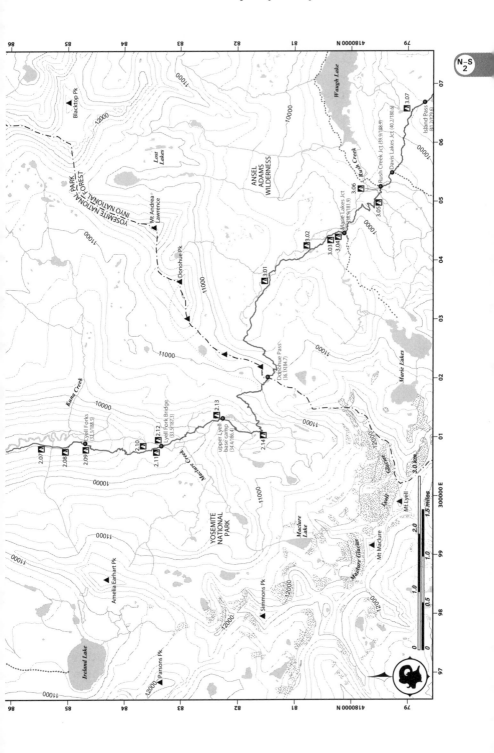

(Continued from page 85)

After another 0.7 mile through similar terrain, the trail and river both curve south–southeast, and the two soon converge. After a brief section of water tumbling across bare rock, you reach Lyell Canyon. You get to enjoy an idyllic scene for the next many miles: The walls of Lyell Canyon rise steeply on either side; the unbelievably clear and often deep, aqua-green waters of the Lyell Fork meander down the middle of the canyon; and flower-filled or yellowing meadows line the edges of the stream. If you are lucky, you will spot a belted king-fisher, with its shrill, cackling call, diving into the water to fish. Your only job is not to disturb the scene for the next party: Be sure to stay on the trail and not trespass into the meadow each time the track becomes a bit deeper or muddier. Two of the flower species you will see through-out Lyell Canyon are the mountain meadow penstemon, with a circular arrangement of 2-centimeter-long, skinny, tubular, purple flowers, and little elephant's head, with an elongated head of 0.5-centimeter-long lavender flowers. If you look at an individual flower upside down, you can see the elephant's ears and trunk. Little elephant's heads are present in nearly every high elevation wet meadow in the Sierra, while the mountain meadow penstemon is sometimes replaced by a quite similar species, the Sierra penstemon; the latter is covered by sticky glands that glow in the sun.

Camping is not allowed in Lyell Canyon until you are 4 miles beyond Tuolumne Meadows, a position approximately marked by a large avalanche path visible on the east canyon wall. While you can always find a few small campsites to the edge of the meadow, the first major camping area is at the junction with the trail to Ireland and Evelyn lakes [8,900' – 4.2/29.4], where there are many campsites just to the northwest of the trail junction. Ireland Creek is easy to wade, or you can work your way across a series of logs to the west of the trail that are often half submerged during high flow. Still with negligible elevation gain, the JMT continues up Lyell Canyon, beneath imposing Potter Point. At several locations where the trail diverges slightly from the river, there are a few campsites to the west of the trail. Enjoy the views, including glances of Mt. Lyell, Yosemite's highest peak, at the head of the canyon, because Lyell Canyon eventually—and quite suddenly—ends. Known as Lyell Forks due to the nearly simultaneous merging of three creeks, it marks the start of the climb out of Lyell Canyon [9,020' – 3.0/32.3]. There is a large campsite soon after you begin the climb.

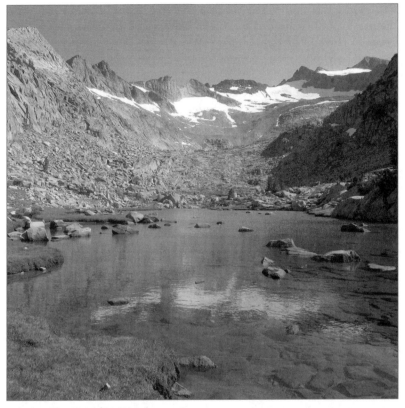

Mt. Lyell and the basin to its northeast

From Lyell Forks, you begin to climb a series of exposed switch-backs, mostly across a slope strewn with old avalanche debris. One of the common shrubs on these disturbed slopes is red elderberry, distinguished by its large leaves, displayed in clusters of seven: The berries are a favorite late-summer food source for wildlife. As you continue climbing, you leave the lodgepole forests that fringe Lyell Canyon and enter stands dominated by mountain hemlocks. The switchbacks end at a forested bench with many campsites. (Note that campfires are prohibited here, even if you find a location just below 9,600 feet!) The trail then crosses the Lyell Fork on a footbridge [9,650′ – 1.1/33.5]; just to the east of the footbridge are two spur trails leading to additional camping. After just a brief pause, the trail resumes its ascent through mixed hemlock and lodgepole forest and past abundant flowers. The slope lessens at an elongate meadow strip that leads to another popular camping area; there are few good campsites and many less-ideal sites used by the latecomers [10,190′ – 0.9/34.4]. The campsites and adjacent lake are fringed by a charming timberline meadow and scattered stands of whitebark pine, the most common timberline species throughout the Sierra; its needles grow in clusters of five, which easily distinguishes it from the two-needled lodgepole pine that grows in the forests below.

If you choose to spend the night here, you will begin your morning with either a chilly wade across the lake near its outlet or with a few easy hops across rocks—if you're lucky—followed by a steep climb up a slope west of the small lake. Numerous trickles cross this slope and the vegetation appears lush until you suddenly level out to the side of a sandy knob. As you round the corner of the knob, look around for a few small, sandy tent sites in the area; additional options are found by walking off-trail to the south; these sites are used mainly by climbers headed to the summit of Mt. Lyell, the imposing 13,114-foot peak to the south. The snowfield you see was once the largest glacier visible from the JMT, but in 2013 it was redesignated as a permanent snow-field, indicating that it no longer has sufficient mass to move downhill. Notably, all current glaciers in the Sierra Nevada formed during the Little Ice Age, a cold period that began 700 years ago. The much larger Pleistocene glaciers had completely disappeared in the interim and the Sierra seems to be heading to another glacier-less period.

Drop down to another creek, which you step across via large rocks. Once across, a short spur trail leads left to a view down the canyon. Meanwhile, the magical presence of the alpine landscape keeps enticing you upward. The views of Mt. Lyell continue to improve as you begin the final climb to Donohue Pass. Alongside rocks, near seasonal streams, you may see the white mountain heather, one of John Muir's favorite flowers. These early-blooming flowers are shaped like little white bells with red caps and can occur in large masses. Also present is the red mountain heather, with more open, red-pink flowers and longer, needle-shaped leaves. Both form mats alongside rocks, although the red heather grows down to lower elevations and has a range that extends farther south in the Sierra. The ascent continues on broken granite slabs and along sandy passageways, delineating fractures in the granite. This makes for engaging, but slightly slower walking as you have to make many tall steps and can't establish an even pace. (Strictly speaking, this rock is granodiorite, a variant of granite with a greater percentage of dark minerals than that found in the Cathedral Range.) Before long, you emerge on the summit of tarn-dotted Donohue Pass [11,060' − 1.7/36.1]. If you wish to climb still higher, a side trip up Donohue Peak or even just the tiny knob north of the pass is recommended (see page 212).

SECTION 3.

Donohue Pass to Island Pass: Rush Creek (5.1 miles)

Donohue Pass delineates the boundary between Yosemite National Park and Ansel Adams Wilderness. To the south you can see Mammoth Mountain and the Mammoth Crest, country you will traverse over the coming days. Excepting the descent from Mt. Whitney, the 5.1-mile leg to the top of Island Pass is the only section of the JMT that is east of the Sierra Crest: Rush Creek drains into Mono Lake, the famous Great Basin salt lake with no outlet. As with the northwest side of the pass, the upper stretch is slow going, for the trail is picking a route down broken slabs and across quite rocky ground. Carefully descending the switchbacks, enjoy the view of the meadow-covered granite basin with abundant glacial erratics—large boulders scattered across the landscape where they were "dumped" by a glacier. The abundance of heath vegetation is an indication of just how wet this area is: Dwarf bilberry, white heather, red heather, and mountain laurel are all common here; mountain laurel has flowers quite similar to red heather, but the plants are spread across flatter, marshier terrain, forming carpets of

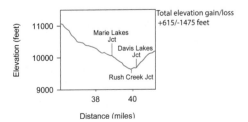

LOCATION	ELEVATION	DISTANCE FROM PREVIOUS POINT	CUMULATIVE DISTANCE	UTM COORDINATES
Donohue Pass	11,060'	—	36.1	11S 302025E 4181480N
Marie Lakes junction	10,050'	2.8	38.9	11S 304468E 4180130N
Rush Creek junction	9,640'	1.0	39.9	11S 305247E 4179506N
Davis Lakes junction	9,690'	0.3	40.2	11S 305493E 4179290N
Island Pass	10,200'	1.0	41.2	11S 306696E 4178711N

plants with larger leaves. There are also the diminutive Rocky Mountain willows crawling along the ground, most easily identifiable if covered by the white fuzz that accompanies their seedpods. Endless small creek crossings may slow your progress in early summer, and the marshy, vegetated ground is mostly too wet and fragile for camping; only a few drier hummocks, denoted by stunted whitebark pine, offer dry, legal, and certainly worthwhile campsites; seek out sandy, previously used sites.

Beyond, your descent alternates between increasingly forested terrain and open, slabby sections, the latter hosting several nice campsites. Before long, you reach the roaring torrent of Rush Creek. A log bridge allows you to cross the flow safely, and just across the stream, you reach the junction with the Marie Lakes Trail [10,050' – 2.8/38.9] to which you can detour for beautiful campsites. You continue your switchbacking descent along the quick-flowing creek and may notice the granite getting darker: You are approaching the boundary between

Panorama south from Donohue Pass

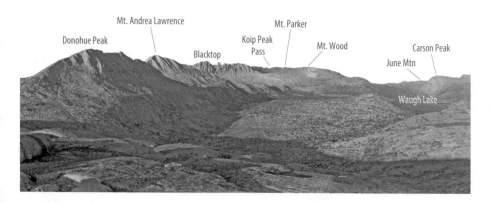

granitic and metamorphosed volcanic rocks, and the granite's chemical composition changes as it approaches the boundary. The trail next reaches an area known as the Rush Creek Forks, named for the many creeks that join together here; the more difficult crossings have log 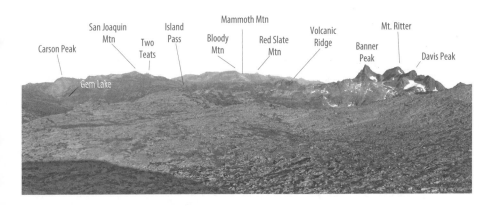 bridges. Along the way, you pass the Rush Creek Trail junction (and access to Waugh Lake), incorrectly marked on the USGS topo maps about 0.15 mile to the north of its current location [9,640' – 1.0/39.9]. You next pass the Davis Lakes junction [9,690' – 0.3/40.2] and begin the climb to Island Pass. The north-facing climb is through dry lodgepole forest with little ground cover, although it's certainly not bare. Pussypaws, which has small balls of pink flowers on short stalks, is one species that tolerates such inhospitable conditions. Its long, skinny, dark green, and slightly succulent leaves hug the ground. The rock here is still the same granodiorite that was found atop Donohue Pass, but within it are inclusions of the metamorphosed volcanic rocks that you will walk through south of Island Pass. (Inclusions is the technical term used when chunks of one rock are embedded within a different type of rock, as often occurs near the boundary or contact between two rock types.) As you approach the summit, the grade lessens and you pass a small tarn with a campsite and walk alongside many seeps colorful with flowers. The climb ends among dry meadows and many lakes and tarns atop Island Pass. Several of these lakes have large populations of mountain yellow-legged frogs. Detour over to have a look, but please refrain from picking them up, for you almost certainly have sunscreen or bug repellent residue on your hands. The unmarked high point is toward the northern end of the plateau [10,200' – 1.0/41.2]. There are many small campsites among the lakes—take a look around.

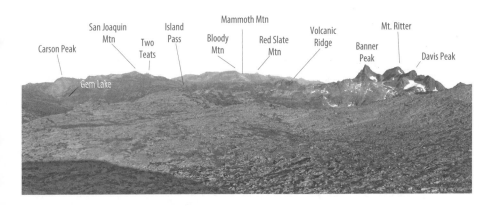

Carson Peak   San Joaquin Mtn   Two Teats   Island Pass   Bloody Mtn   Mammoth Mtn   Red Slate Mtn   Volcanic Ridge   Banner Peak   Mt. Ritter   Davis Peak   Gem Lake

SECTION 4.

Island Pass to Madera–Fresno County Line: Middle Fork of the San Joaquin River (22.8 miles)

From now until you reach the summit of Mt. Whitney, the JMT again lies on the west side of the crest: All water drains into the San Joaquin Valley. For 85 miles, you will be in the drainage area of the San Joaquin River, whose waters eventually flow into the San Francisco Bay. You will first descend the main Middle Fork drainage, then ascend the Fish Creek drainage, cross Mono Creek and Bear Creek, and finally enter the main South Fork drainage that you follow to Muir Pass. But of more interest to you now is the sweeping view of the dark Ritter Range, of which Banner Peak stands out most prominently. Those dark rocks likely resulted from a catastrophic caldera collapse 100 million years ago; the magma that erupted was some of the same molten rock that formed the plutons deep underground. The volcanic rock was then metamorphosed during the tectonic events that led to the continued formation of the underlying granite.

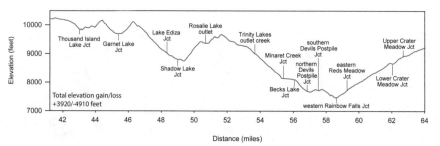

LOCATION	ELEVATION	DISTANCE FROM PREVIOUS POINT	CUMULATIVE DISTANCE	UTM COORDINATES
Island Pass	10,200'	—	41.2	11S 306696E 4178711N
Thousand Island Lake junction	9,830'	1.8	43.0	11S 308733E 4177711N
Garnet Lake junction	9,690'	2.4	45.4	11S 310473E 4176161N
Lake Ediza junction	9,000'	2.9	48.3	11S 311074E 4173429N
Shadow Lake junction	8,780'	0.7	49.0	11S 311695E 4173755N
Rosalie Lake outlet	9,350'	1.7	50.7	11S 313013E 4173125N
Trinity Lakes outlet crossing	8,990'	3.0	53.7	11S 314766E 4170105N
Minaret Creek junction (Johnston Meadow)	8,120'	1.7	55.4	11S 314836E 4168536N
Beck Lakes junction	8,080'	0.7	56.1	11S 315344E 4167773N
northern Devils Postpile junction	7,680'	0.7	56.8	11S 315738E 4166946N
southern Devils Postpile junction	7,710'	0.7	57.5	11S 315861E 4165921N
western Rainbow Falls junction	7,460'	1.1	58.6	11S 316246E 4164827N
western Reds Meadow junction	7,640'	0.6	59.2	11S 316792E 4164496N
eastern Reds Meadow junction	7,710'	0.1	59.3	11S 316898E 4164358N
lower Crater Meadow junction (Mammoth Pass)	8,650'	2.7	62.0	11S 318340E 4162258N
upper Crater Meadow junction	8,910'	0.7	62.7	11S 318941E 4161689N
Madera–Fresno County Line	9,210'	1.3	64.0	11S 319942E 4160144N

N–S 4

You descend dry slopes toward Thousand Island Lake, whose surface is dotted with dozens of rocky islets. Although dry, the volcanic soils sport an amazing diversity of wildflowers—including a patch of periwinkle-colored western blue flax, a species you will not see again until you ascend the slopes of Mt. Whitney, and large masses of mountain prettyfaces, which are pale yellow, six-petaled flowers related to

(Continued on page 98)

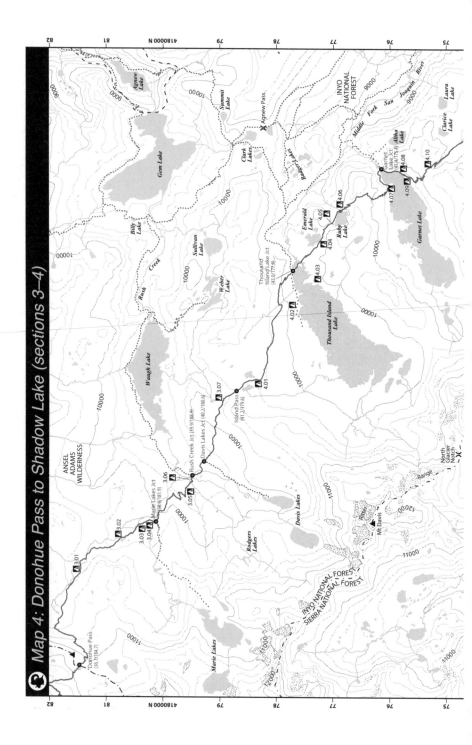

Map 4: Donohue Pass to Shadow Lake (sections 3–4)

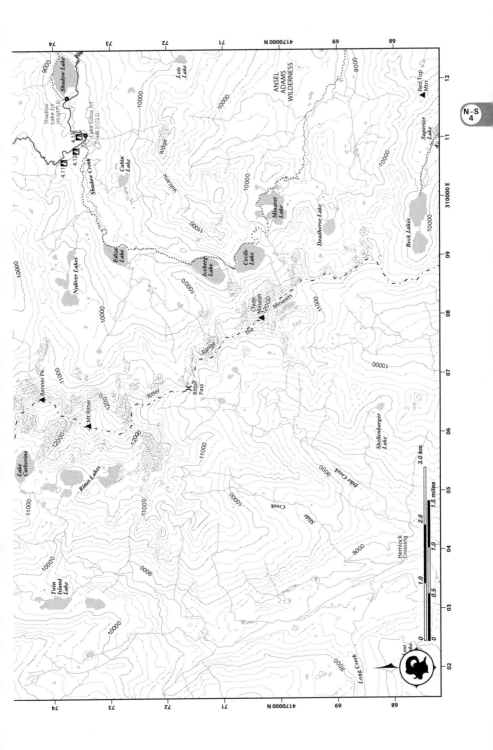

(Continued from page 95)

lilies. Bright blue mountain bluebirds are commonly seen on these bare slopes, perched on snags between insect-catching forays. As the descent levels out, you reach a junction with a trail that leads around the lake's northwest shore, where there are many camping options. Note that camping is prohibited within 0.25 mile of the lake's outlet. Views of Banner Peak over Thousand Island Lake are irresistible for photographers and were memorialized in many of Ansel Adams's most famous photographs—how appropriate that this area is now part of his namesake wilderness. A few more steps bring you to a junction where the JMT and the Pacific Crest Trail (PCT), which have been one and the same since Tuolumne Meadows, diverge for several miles [9,830' – 1.8/43.0]. A fork of this trail later heads to the Clark Lakes, Agnew Lake, and the Rush Creek Trailhead (see Appendix A).

You head southeast on a footbridge over the outlet of Thousand Island Lake, noting additional campsites on the bluff to the southwest of the lake, and make a moderate climb past pretty Emerald Lake. (The northern half of this lake is still within the camping exclusion zone.) You continue upward to stark, deep Ruby Lake, surrounded on the west by impressive walls, and to the northeast by enormous mats of manzanita. There are small campsites near the outlet, beneath mountain hemlock cover. The JMT climbs again, to the ridgetop above Ruby Lake, before descending on rocky switchbacks to beautiful, windy Garnet Lake, another splendid islet-dotted lake. Note that, as with Thousand Island Lake, camping is prohibited within a quarter mile of Garnet Lake's outlet. Fortunately, near the bottom of the switchbacks, you find a junction with a use trail that leads to campsites on Garnet's northwest shore; you immediately reach a large site, but more secluded options are available the farther you detour toward Garnet's head. While only Banner Peak was visible from Thousand Island Lake, both Mt. Ritter and Banner Peak are now prominent. You trace Garnet's north shore briefly, passing steep metamorphic bluffs and large patches of red heather, cross its outlet on a footbridge, and immediately pass a junction with a rough trail that descends northeast into the canyon of the Middle Fork of the San Joaquin River and one route to Agnew Meadows [9,690' – 2.4/45.4].

The JMT now traverses upward along Garnet's south shore, passing through wet streamside vegetation that includes the bright red-flowered great red paintbrush. Paintbrushes have elongated heads of very narrow, tubular, beaked blossoms, and the great red paintbrush is the tallest of the many Sierra species. It is also the only one to prefer

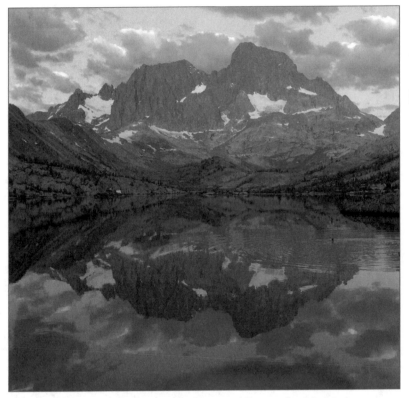

Sunrise over Garnet Lake with Mt. Ritter and Banner Peak behind

stream banks and seeps. You pass a few more campsites perched on small flats to the side of the lake, as well as sites close to the lakeshore below. Beyond, the trail turns southeast to climb steeply up the ridge south of Garnet Lake. Halfway up, near a giant mountain hemlock, are tufts of bell-shaped, light pink alumroot emerging from cracks in the rock; they are common, growing alongside shaded rock walls throughout the Sierra. At a saddle atop the ridge, there are few mediocre tent sites and a swimming-pool-size pond that warms up enough by midsummer for pleasant bathing—or you may find it dry.

You now begin a 1,100-foot descent, past a small meadow and through a tiny canyon with a mixed lodgepole pine and mountain hemlock cover. The two-tone needles of the latter always stand out: The young needles are a much brighter green than the old foliage. Also apparent, the branch tips droop downward, for the young shoots are

(Continued on page 102)

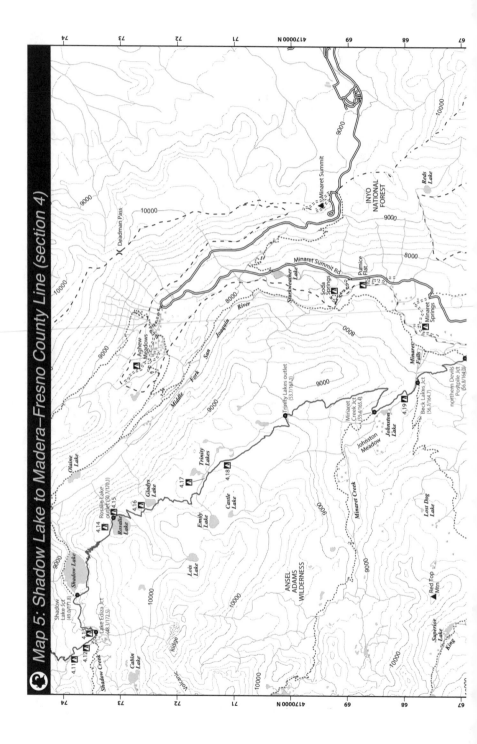

Map 5: Shadow Lake to Madera–Fresno County Line (section 4)

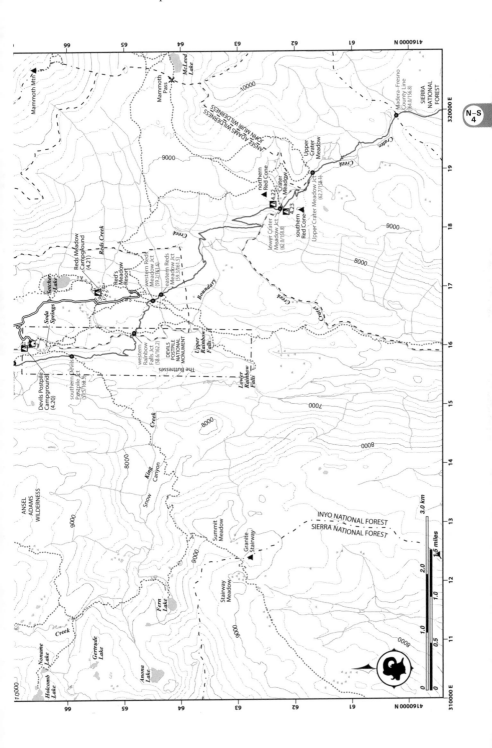

(Continued from page 99)

weak. A few western white pines, with their larger cones, are also present; look closely at the beautiful cone scales, which have a vibrant pattern of light and dark brown. At a distinct bend in the trail is the junction with the unmarked and unmaintained trail to Laura Lake. Before long, you emerge on a dry knob with a majestic western juniper, an understory of manzanita, and an excellent view of the Minarets, the skyline of spires to the south of Mt. Ritter. You reenter the forest and soon converge with a tributary of Shadow Creek and pass shady flats with good campsites. Next, you reach a T-junction: A right turn takes you to Ediza Lake, while the JMT turns east (left) toward Shadow Lake and Agnew Meadows [9,000' – 3.0/48.3]. Just beyond is a single campsite to the north of the trail, the last good site until Rosalie Lake, for camping is prohibited between the river and the trail between this junction and Shadow Lake as well as near Shadow Lake's shores.

You alternately descend through lodgepole forest and across open, slabby knobs, still composed of metavolcanic rock. The fast-flowing stream is a good location to spot an American dipper, also known as a water ouzel—a round, grayish bird that can often be seen diving in and out of rapids in search of insects; its constantly bending knees confirm its identity. Upstream of the Shadow Lake inlet, you reach another junction: Straight ahead takes you down to the Middle Fork of the San Joaquin River and out to Agnew Meadows, while the JMT turns south (right) across a handsome footbridge [8,780' – 0.7/49.0].

After skirting the south shore of Shadow Lake, the trail continues south. The elevation profile certainly indicates there is a long climb ahead, but do not be too discouraged, as the switchbacks are well-graded and the dense hemlock forest will provide long stretches of shade. A little more than 650 feet later, you reach a small saddle and briefly emerge from the forest before descending to shady Rosalie Lake. There are mountain hemlocks overhead and poisonous western Labrador tea underfoot as you cross the outlet on a logjam [9,350' – 1.7/50.7]. The latter resembles an azalea, and indeed the two are in the same genus. There are some nice campsites nearby.

You skirt Rosalie's north and east shores before climbing a little and then dipping down to mountain hemlock-fringed Gladys Lake, which also has a number of good campsites. After passing Gladys Lake, the JMT rolls over a little saddle and begins a long, gradual descent of Volcanic Ridge, still under mountain hemlocks, western white pines, and a few lodgepole pines. As you continue, you will notice increasing numbers of downed trees, including big gaps where there was once dense forest. You

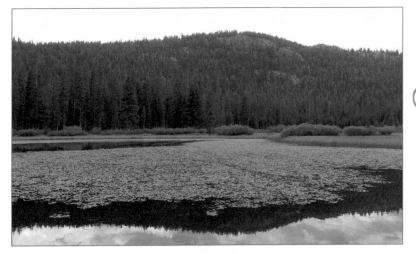

Johnston Lake

are entering the area decimated by the November 30, 2011, Devils Windstorm that toppled more than 10,000 trees between Yosemite and Tully Hole. This extreme event brought sustained 125–150 mph winds from the north–northeast. While most winter storms come from the west, funneling winds up-valley, these were northern winds and roared down-canyon. The trees along the Middle Fork of the San Joaquin had roots well buttressed to withstand the southerly winds, but not those from the north. Over the coming days you will again and again pass downed trees and walk in the sun where there was once shade.

You pass the attractive, marshy Trinity Lakes, a series of shallow ponds strung out along the trail. If you are willing to walk a few hundred feet to water, there are many sandy campsites on the west side of the trail, but also keep your eyes peeled for campsites closer to water. The JMT skirts Lower Trinity Lake and then crosses the creek draining Trinity Lakes [8,990' – 3.0/53.7], which features a colorful display of wildflowers, including crimson columbine, with bright, red-orange flowers that point upright and five long spurs that dangle behind. Note that this creek may be dry during late season. This forest is at a lower elevation than many others along the JMT, and is filled with birdlife: Keep your ears open for a black-backed woodpecker whacking on a dead tree or a northern goshawk screeching as it flies through the forest.

Both the angle of the slope and the angle of your descent now increase, the slope becomes drier, and the vegetation changes. For the first time since Sunrise Creek, you encounter red fir, mixed with continued western white pines and a few lodgepole pines. Although you

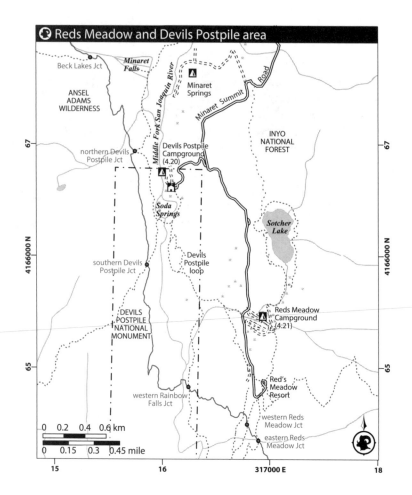

only rarely see an outcrop, the bedrock deep beneath your feet is again granite, not the metavolcanic rocks you have been walking through since Thousand Island Lake. Overlying, and hiding, the solid rock is pumice sand, undoubtedly mixed with some decaying granite. The dry slope is dotted with red-colored rose thistles and aromatic lavender-colored pennyroyal, a mint, but occasionally you cross a small seep and encounter a wetter plant community. Just north of Johnston Meadow, you reach a T-junction with a trail that goes northwest to Minaret Lake, while the JMT heads left (southeast) toward Devils Postpile [8,120' – 1.7/55.4]. Across the trail are boggy Johnston Meadow and little Johnston Lake.

The JMT continues descending over loose pumice, passing a small campsite northwest of the trail and just beyond reaching a crossing of Minaret Creek on a log bridge. This enticing, pebble-bottomed creek is a wonderful place to cool your feet. You shortly pass a junction with trail west to Beck Lakes [8,080' – 0.7/56.1] and continue down a granite slope that is, again, mostly overlaid by pumice sand. Many of the tallest trees on this descent were toppled by the windstorm; imagine standing in the valley as these trees fell one after another. Beyond, and just inside the boundary of Devils Postpile National Monument, you reach a large X-junction [7,680' – 0.8/56.8]. At this point, the PCT, coming in from the northeast, rejoins the JMT.

Although the JMT continues along the southwestern (right) branch of the X-junction, if you have not previously visited Devils Postpile, I recommend a detour to this geologic attraction, since the JMT provides only fleeting and distant glances of the structure. Others may take the junction to Devils Postpile to find camping for the night or to access Mammoth Lakes. There are campgrounds at both Devils Postpile and near the Red's Meadow Resort, a short distance to the south, although only at Reds Meadow are there showers and a site specially reserved for backpackers. Both locations also provide access to the shuttle bus, which runs every 20 minutes midsummer and travels to the Mammoth Mountain ski area, your "gateway" to the town of Mammoth Lakes. (On the opposite page, see the map of the Devils Postpile and Reds Meadow areas.)

To reach Devils Postpile, take the southeast-trending fork down to the riverbank, where you soon find a bridge. Cross the bridge and continue south to a short, sign-posted loop around the postpile. A bit of geologic background: Devils Postpile formed less than 100,000 years ago, following an eruption of basaltic magma. Slow, even cooling conditions and magma with a consistent chemical composition throughout allowed the hexagonal columns to form. Because of the topography, an unusually deep flow of magma accumulated, such that the interior was well-insulated and cooled slowly and evenly. As magma cools, it contracts and hence must fracture. Physics dictates that fractures 120 degrees apart most efficiently release building stress, leading to hexagonal columns. Devils Postpile is one of the world's tallest and most nearly perfect examples of columnar basalt. Be sure to walk around the loop, which takes you both to the top of the formation, where glacially polished tops of columns are exposed, and to the base of the formation, where you can gaze up at the columns and gawk at the talus field of hexagonal-shaped rocks. From the southern end of this short loop, follow the trail that leads to Reds Meadow. At the next junction, bear left and, a short distance later, bend to the right; this trail will cross roads twice and then reach the Red's Meadow Resort. If you instead turn right at the junction beyond the loop, you will more quickly rejoin the JMT but have a longer route to Reds Meadow.

To bypass Devils Postpile, take the upper, south-trending fork and climb gently up a dusty track across a steep, pumice slope. With the exception of one knob, the postpiles are hidden from view. You pass a second X-junction, where another trail from Devils Postpile crosses the JMT and heads southwest toward King Creek [7,710' – 0.7/57.5]. The JMT continues to the southeast (left). Shortly after this junction, you enter a burn area, the result of a large, lightning-caused forest fire in 1992, named the Rainbow Fire. Although young trees dot the landscape, it will be many years before this area is again a forest. The dusty pumice substrate might be unappealing, but the open slopes display abundant bird life, including yellow-rumped warblers, mountain bluebirds, and swallows, as well as a community of plants that only thrive following burns. You will walk past abundant Sierra gooseberries with 1-centimeter-wide, spiny (but tasty if you suck out the insides) berries; mountain whitethorn, a shrub with intimidating thorns and small, blue-green leaves; and scarlet penstemon, with its stalk full of bright red, tubular flowers. After curving down and traversing a wet meadow, you cross the Middle Fork of the San Joaquin on a footbridge and almost immediately reach a junction [7,460' – 1.1/58.6]. From either this point or the next junction, you can detour south to Rainbow Falls if you have the time and energy.

Over the next 0.5 mile, you pass three more junctions as the JMT heads east and skirts to the south of the Red's Meadow Resort. The first leads to the Rainbow Falls trailhead (and bus stop), while the second [7,640' – 0.5/59.2] and third [7,710' – 0.1/59.3] provide accesses to the Red's Meadow Resort, where you may have a food parcel to retrieve, wish to eat at the café, take a shower, fill your water bottles, buy additional supplies, or find a campground for the night (see page 23 for details). Continuing on the JMT, you ascend yet another pumice trail, still in the area denuded by the Rainbow Fire. If you find yourself annoyed by its dusty nature, stop and appreciate how soft it is underfoot! As before, the wildflower displays can be astonishing and the aerial antics of the abundant swallows engaging. And as you stare at the thick, spiny shrubs on either side of the trail, you'll be thankful to be on a maintained trail. Camping is impractical along this stretch of the JMT due to the dense undergrowth, and you must reach Crater Creek by nightfall. As you climb, you first cross four branches of Boundary Creek and slowly, as the slope becomes steeper, enter areas with more standing trees—Jeffrey pines, western junipers, western white pines, and white firs. In the distance, you can see the outline of the two Red Cones. Many switchbacks later, you find yourself at the base of the northern Red Cone, at a junction with a little-used trail northeast to Mammoth

Pass [8,650' – 2.8/62.0]. Just beyond this point, you cross Crater Creek on a fallen log. Along the stream banks, a short distance below the crossing, a few, mostly collapsed lava tubes are visible. Among the many fallen logs, there are a few small campsites on the south side of Crater Creek and one a short distance up the northern Red Cone.

An ascent of one (or both) of the Red Cones is highly recommended (see page 213). The vista from the summits not only lets you gaze over the country you've covered since Donohue Pass, but you also get a close-up view of Mammoth Mountain. A bit of geologic history: The volcanic activity of the last 3 million years formed the pumice deposits you have walked over and will continue to walk over. About 760,000 years ago, an enormous eruption formed Long Valley Caldera, a bit east of the Sierra, depositing ash as far east as Nebraska. At 220,000 years, Mammoth Mountain, a dormant volcano, is a more recent addition. The Red Cones themselves are less than 10,000 years old. These events are separate from the much older volcanic events that led to the formation of rocks that make up the Ritter Range. Today Mammoth Mountain is best known as a vast ski area that receives enormous quantities of snow. This is no coincidence, as the passes that cross the Sierra Crest in this vicinity are the lowest for a great distance north and south, allowing storms that are elsewhere blocked by tall mountains to funnel straight to the slopes of Mammoth. Its founder, who had previously worked as a snow surveyor, had done his homework.

From the junction with Mammoth Pass, you continue south up a small ravine and cross Crater Creek again. Abundant wet meadow wildflowers grow on and near the moist stream banks, including several species forming mats along the ground, such as carpet clover, which has small, white flowers, and primrose monkeyflower, which has single, yellow, tubular flowers attached atop 2- to 4-inch stalks. It is always identifiable by its light green leaves pressed flat to the ground and long hairs that hold the morning dew, causing the plants to glow in the sun. As you continue south along the JMT, these species will become familiar faces in wet alpine meadows or at the borders of little seeps. The next junction also leads to Mammoth Pass [8,910' – 0.7/62.7]; to reach the pass, head right at a second fork just beyond the JMT.

Skirting to the west of Upper Crater Meadow, the JMT crunches south–southeast over pumice, crossing a small fork of Crater Creek, and then crossing Crater Creek itself again. This gradual ascent ends approximately 0.2 mile after the last creek crossing, atop a sandy saddle and unlikely drainage divide. This point, the Madera–Fresno County Line, marks the boundary between the main Middle Fork of the San Joaquin drainage and Fish Creek [9,210' – 1.3/64.0].

SECTION 5.

Madera–Fresno County Line to Silver Pass: Fish Creek Fork of the Middle Fork of the San Joaquin River (17.7 miles)

From the drainage divide, the JMT continues through open lodgepole forest. It drops a little, passes an indistinct and unmarked junction with a lateral up Deer Creek, and then fords Deer Creek [9,100' – 1.0/65.0], near which are a number of campsites frequented by parties with livestock. Fill your water bottles at Deer Creek, for the next reliable water is at Duck Creek, nearly 6 miles away. To many, the next section is among the most monotonous on the JMT: Until you approach the Duck Pass junction, the vegetation and views change little. But pay close attention to a change in rock type, as you are still on pumice substrate initially, but will transition to walking on granitic gravel as you climb gradually along the north wall of Cascade Valley. At first, the forest contains a mixture

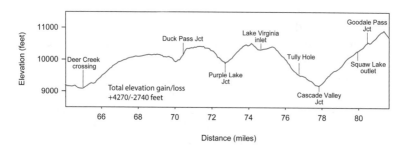

LOCATION	ELEVATION	DISTANCE FROM PREVIOUS POINT	CUMULATIVE DISTANCE	UTM COORDINATES
Madera–Fresno County Line	9,210'	—	64.0	11S 319942E 4160144N
Deer Creek	9,100'	1.0	65.0	11S 320460E 4159139N
Duck Pass junction	10,160'	5.5	70.5	11S 326107E 4156217N
Purple Lake trail junction	9,940'	2.2	72.7	11S 327817E 4154979N
Lake Virginia inlet crossing	10,330'	2.0	74.7	11S 329263E 4153696N
Tully Hole (McGee Pass junction)	9,540'	2.1	76.8	11S 329961E 4152066N
Cascade Valley (Fish Creek) junction	9,190'	1.1	77.9	11S 329202E 4150912N
Squaw Lake outlet	10,290'	2.1	80.0	11S 329933E 4149416N
Goodale Pass junction	10,540'	0.5	80.5	11S 329463E 4149123N
Silver Pass	10,740'	1.2	81.7	11S 330013E 4148295N

N–S
5

of lodgepole and western white pines, but the western white pines disappear before long, as only lodgepole pines can survive under the dry conditions dictated by the southern exposure and coarse volcanic soils. The ground, likewise, is nearly bare—most notable are a few species in the mustard family, whose flowers are distinguished by a four-pronged arrangement resembling a cross: sanddune wallflower, with its heads of many yellow flowers on a tall stalk, and several types of rockcress, with small, white to purple flowers on a slightly shorter stem. By midsummer, most individual plants no longer have flowers and are instead decorated by long seedpods; species of rockcress are distinguished by the width of the pods and whether they are upright or drooping. Rocky slopes sport a few shrubs, including mountain big sagebrush, manzanita, and a relative of oaks, bush chinquapin, whose leaf undersides are gold-colored and whose fruits are round prickly balls. Openings in the forest provide occasional glimpses south to the Silver Divide. Among the many birds you are likely to see in this area are the red-breasted nuthatches, circling down a tree trunk in search of insects and "honking" like a truck backing up; the ubiquitous dark-eyed junco, a large sparrow with a dark head and streaks of white on its tail; and blue grouse. The trail sidles in and

(Continued on page 112)

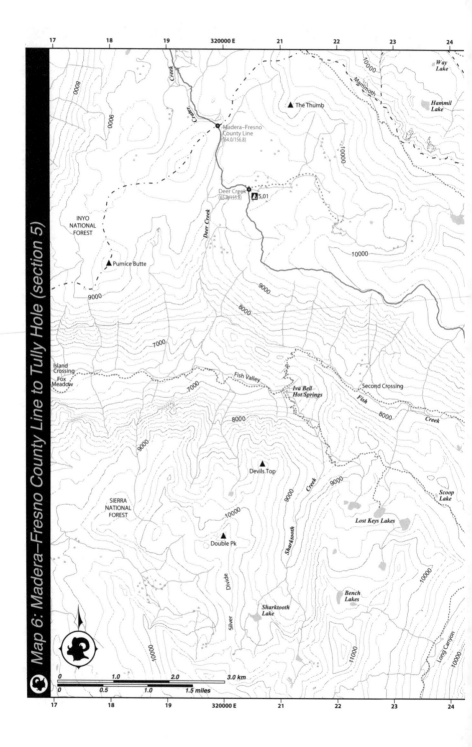

17   18   19   320000 E   21   22   23   24

Way Lake

Mammoth

Hammil Lake

▲ The Thumb

Madera–Fresno County Line (64.0/156.8)

Deer Creek (65.0/155.8)   ▲ 5.01

INYO NATIONAL FOREST

Deer Creek

10000

9000

▲ Pumice Butte

9000

8000

7000

Island Crossing
Fox Meadow

Fish Valley

Iva Bell Hot Springs

Second Crossing

Fish Creek

8000

▲ Devils Top

Sharktooth Creek

Scoop Lake

Lost Keys Lakes

SIERRA NATIONAL FOREST

10000

▲ Double Pk

Divide

Silver

Sharktooth Lake

Bench Lakes

Long Canyon

0   1.0   2.0   3.0 km
0   0.5   1.0   1.5 miles

17   18   19   320000 E   21   22   23   24

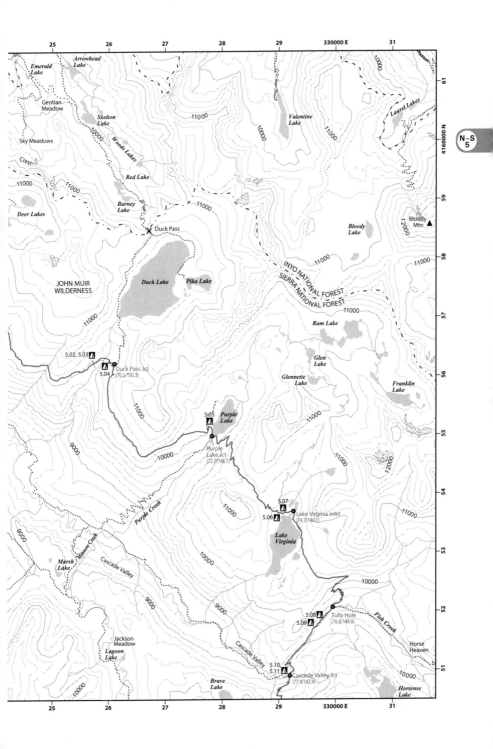

(Continued from page 109)

out of several side valleys, minimizing elevation change, en route to the Duck Creek drainage. Toward the end of this long, ascending traverse, you cross onto granite, at last leaving the pumice behind. After a few days of the foot-pounding granite cobble and gravel, you might even begin to miss the dusty but soft pumice sand. Eventually, the trail angles into the valley of Duck Creek and you make an easy descent to a handful of small campsites clustered among granite slabs near the western side of the crossing. Follow the creek bank downstream to find additional sites. The ford across Duck Creek is not dangerous, but under high water it is a likely wade. A little beyond the creek, the JMT begins a steep switch-backing climb past a junction with a trail to Duck Lake and Duck Pass [10,160' – 5.5/70.5]. Did you notice that the creek crossing and junction are back in dark metavolcanic rocks? You traverse across the boundary between granitic and metavolcanic rocks several times between here and Lake Virginia; see how many contacts you can find.

From the junction, your ascent continues out of the Duck Creek valley and back around to a southern exposure. Here, there are fewer trees, and, in places, you have a beautiful view of the walls of glaciated Cascade Valley and southeast toward Mt. Abbot, a peak on the Sierra Crest. Although it is dry, many flowers dot the granite soil. You may have seen two earlier: the wavyleaf paintbrush and shaggy hawkweed. The paintbrush, a dominant species on all dry slopes, sports a dense head of red-orange tubular flowers and is distinguished from the many other paintbrushes by its wavy-margined leaves. The hawkweed has small yellow flowers that look like miniature dandelions, and its leaves are covered in long white hairs. Pennyroyal and mountain pride pen-stemon are also common here. Before long, you reach a use trail that leads to the west shore of beautiful Purple Lake; in the past there were many campsites here, but many have been at least temporarily obliter-ated by the 2011 blowdown. The JMT continues toward Purple Lake's outlet, passing a junction that leads down into Cascade Valley [9,940' – 2.3/72.7], before crossing on a stout bridge. Camping is prohibited within 300 feet of the outlet.

Now the JMT makes a dry, switchbacking climb to the ridge east of Purple Lake, before leveling out as you approach a wide saddle. Near the summit, spreading carpets of Sierra arnica grace some of the slopes. These large yellow flowers, related to sunflowers, appear sporadically in the open lodgepole forests. Nearer the saddle is a community of dry-site subalpine and alpine species. Large patches of long-stemmed, five-petaled white flowers with mousetail-like stalks of leaves may stand

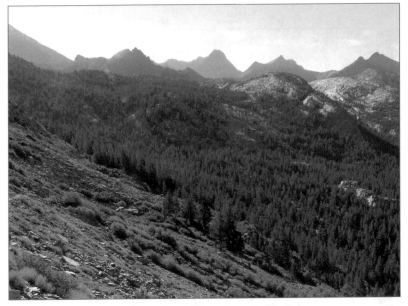

Descending to Tully Hole with the Sierra Crest behind

out—Sierra mousetail. Steep walls and talus fields greet you at the summit, the first time you have encountered such landscape on your southward journey. The pile of rock just to the south of the trail is not a moraine, but a rock glacier, a large mound of talus, likely with ice in its core and slowly moving downslope. The ice at the center of rock glaciers might even be older than the Sierra's ice glaciers—if only there were an easy way to core into it. As you travel farther south, rock glaciers will become common features.

You now descend to Lake Virginia [10,330' – 2.0/74.7], a lovely, large subalpine lake with open views to the south and colorful meadows along its northern shore. Particularly striking are two more species of paintbrush to add to your growing palette, the purple Lemmon's paintbrush and the red and yellow Peirson's paintbrush. Like the two species you have seen previously, these paintbrushes have dense heads of pointed tubular flowers, but only these two species of paintbrush occur in such enormous masses, coloring entire meadows in all but the driest years. There are campsites among scattered trees, both to the southwest of the trail as you approach the lake, and on the sandy knob to the northwest of the lake. As you leave the lake, stop in the first stand

(Continued on page 116)

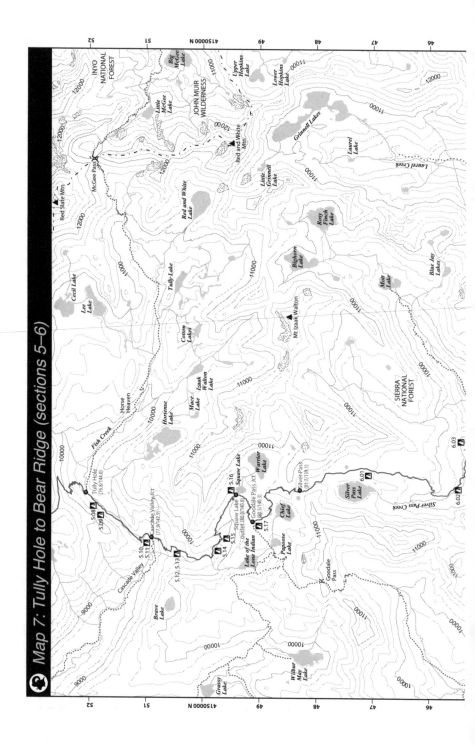

Map 7: Tully Hole to Bear Ridge (sections 5–6)

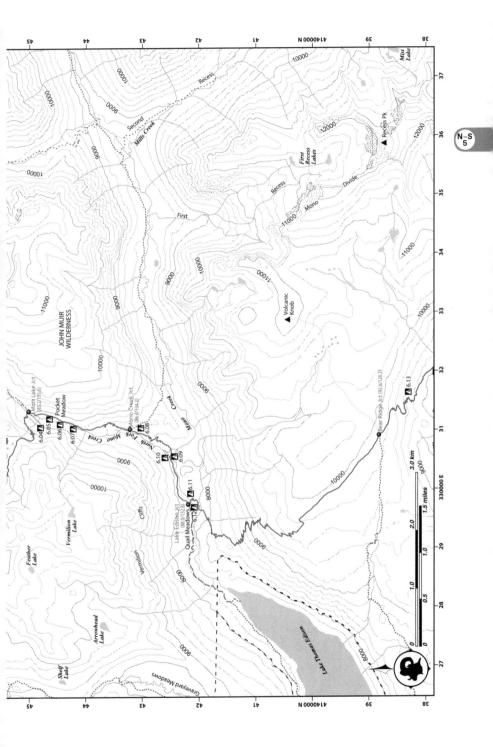

(Continued from page 113)

of lodgepole pines—you might be lucky and see some mountain chick-adees up close. The little birds turn upside-down as they feed and, here, the trees have some low branches. You can always tell when these birds are nearby by their "chick-a-dee-dee" call; one higher, shorter note, followed by two lower, longer ones.

From Lake Virginia, the trail climbs gradually upward and curves southeast over a broad, sandy saddle before switchbacking down a steep, dry slope toward Tully Hole. The verdant meadow around Tully Hole and the lovely headwaters of the Fish Creek drainage look enticing from above—and since you are still above the mosquitoes, you can enjoy the view without the annoyance of the bugs below. As you descend the switchbacks, you will note that this seemingly desolate, dry, sandy slope is alive with an enormous diversity of flowers. Lower down the slope, the ends of each switchback approach little streams and the denser vegetation that grows where water is abundant. One beautiful wet-site plant is Coulter's fleabane daisy, a white daisy with many exquisitely narrow ray petals. Another is Kelley's tiger lily, boasting a tall stalk, sometimes heavily laden with beautiful orange flowers featuring curled-back petals. The 2011 blowdown has changed the landscape around Tully Hole as well, with logs now covering a large stock camp. Beyond is the junction with the trail that crosses Fish Creek to climb eastward up to McGee Pass [9,540' – 2.1/76.8].

Meanwhile, the JMT descends impressive Fish Creek, passing beautiful sections of slab and deep swimming holes, as well as a few barely flat campsites. Before long, you emerge from the lodgepole forest onto a steep slope with picturesque western junipers dotting the rocky bluffs.

Panorama north from Silver Pass; photographed by Nick Knight

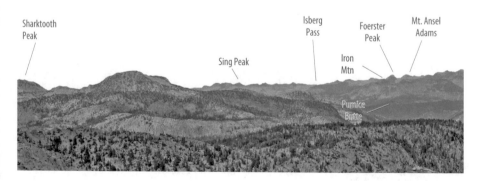

The trail switchbacks down to reach Fish Creek, which you safely cross on a steel footbridge. The three-petaled, mostly white flowers of the Leichtlin's mariposa lily dot these slopes; *mariposa* is the Spanish word for "butterfly," and the petals of many mariposa lilies indeed look like brightly colored wings. After the stream crossing, you enter the first diverse conifer forest since Deer Creek. You pass one campsite shortly before a small creek crossing and a second on a knob just before the Cascade Valley junction [9,190' – 1.1/77.9]. The trail junction, nestled among old avalanche debris, is not always obviously marked, so make sure you take the left fork that begins the climb up to Silver Pass. This junction may be particularly confusing because many maps, including the USGS 7.5-minute topos, show the junction farther downstream.

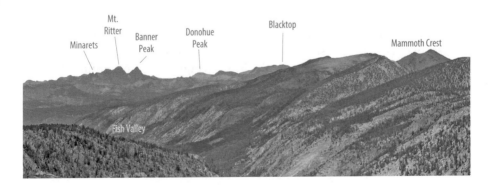

The JMT turns southeast here and begins ascending toward Silver Pass along the east side of the creek. You are traveling through a dense hemlock and lodgepole forest. The thick tree cover feels odd in the Sierra, where you nearly always have a filtered view through the trees. Occasional benches to the west of the trail provide small campsites, ringed by heath vegetation: Labrador tea, dwarf bilberries, and red mountain heather are common in the understory. Black-eyed juncos and American robin, a species of thrush with a burnt red belly, are likely present around the tree bases. Around 9,700 feet, you emerge from this magical forest and cross the creek twice in rapid succession, once at a lupine-covered crossing and thereafter on a footbridge in front of a beautiful little marshy meadow. There are a few campsites among open trees just southeast of the crossing.

As you resume your upward journey on a relatively steep trail, the forest becomes thinner and drier. You skirt around to the south-facing side of the ravine, noting only stunted trees and vegetation of dry, sub-alpine, granite slopes. Many of the species were also abundant at lower elevations, while others will become ever more common as you approach the higher passes to the south. At these elevations, Clark's nutcrackers, relatives of the jays, are common and noisy. These light gray-and-black birds feed predominately on whitebark pine nuts and congregate at upper elevations in late summer. Most amazing is their natural history: They hide many of the pine nuts they harvest, burying them on the surrounding slopes; they can memorize the locations of up to 10,000 nuts. They then sustain themselves through the winter by eating from the large stashes. They are clever enough to hide the nuts on a diversity of slope aspects, ensuring a continuous supply as the snow melts. Because they breed in March, you will never see the young—unless you are on skis.

Alongside a rock outcrop, you may note a succulent with small yellow starlike flowers, Sierra stonecrop. One of the common shrubs on this slope, ocean spray, boasts dense heads of white, five-petaled flowers on pinkish stems and small, serrate leaves. The colorful shrubs bloom for much of the summer. The trail levels out at small Squaw Lake, which is surrounded by alpine meadows and steep cliffs of light-colored granite, very different from the dark, imposing cliffs you have admired since Island Pass [10,290' – 2.1/80.0]. A few sandy, exposed campsites are to the northwest of its outlet, which you cross on large, solid rocks.

From Squaw Lake, you climb briefly and then level out at a junction with the trail from Goodale Pass [10,540' – 0.5/80.5]. The JMT heads south–southeast (left) to skirt dramatic Chief Lake. You are now just about at timberline: Stunted whitebark pines still dot the landscape, but the ground cover is dominated by low-growing alpine species. Frosted wild buckwheat, a common species down into montane forest, forms large mats and is easily identified by its small, fuzzy leaves and ball-like heads of minute yellow flowers that turn red as they go to seed. There are a few sandy, exposed campsites among the tarns north of Chief Lake and also, when water is available, to the left side of the trail as you approach the pass. Through much of the season, there may be a small but quite steep snowbank as you ascend to a shoulder just before Silver Pass. Once the snow melts it is decorated with beautiful little white and pink flowers: Tolmie's saxifrage, a species that grows only on sandy slopes that hold late snow. When you reach the high point, look closely at the landscape and you will realize that you are not yet on the drainage divide or the official pass. You won't enter the Mono Creek drainage until after you have descended the first two switchbacks [10,740' – 1.2/81.7].

SECTION 6.

Silver Pass to Selden Pass:
Mono and Bear Creeks (20.0 miles)

A long these next miles of the JMT, you will travel the farthest from the Sierra Crest and often at lower elevations. Be sure to enjoy the expansive forests, as they will become sparser as you head south and higher. But now you should enjoy the excellent view south, where you can observe much of your route to the top of Selden Pass. Seven Gables is one of the most dramatic peaks, and its sub-peak, to the west, has the seven namesake gables or ridges, running longitudinally down its north face. As you descend the sandy trail, note that the vegetation is different on the warmer, southern side of the pass. Approaching Silver Pass Lake, you walk alternately across stretches of alpine meadow and open, sandy flats. The latter are inhabited by Belding's ground squirrels resembling miniature groundhogs in shape and in behavior as they stand upright and stare at you from their burrow entrances. The JMT curves eastward, away from Silver Pass Lake, but if you wish to camp

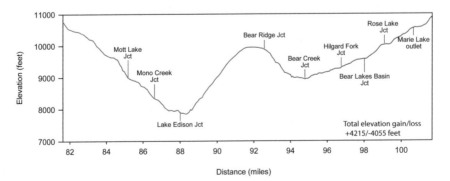

LOCATION	ELEVATION	DISTANCE FROM PREVIOUS POINT	CUMULATIVE DISTANCE	UTM COORDINATES
Silver Pass	10,740'	—	81.7	11S 330013E 4148295N
Mott Lake junction	8,990'	3.5	85.2	11S 331344E 4145016N
Mono Creek junction	8,350'	1.4	86.6	11S 331025E 4143220N
Lake Edison (Quail Meadows) junction	7,900'	1.4	88.0	11S 329749E 4142183N
Bear Ridge junction	9,870'	4.6	92.6	11S 330920E 4138825N
Bear Creek junction	8,940'	2.2	94.8	11S 332846E 4137180N
Hilgard Fork junction	9,320'	2.0	96.8	11S 333894E 4134670N
Bear Lakes Basin junction	9,580'	1.2	98.0	11S 334658E 4132945N
Three Island Lake junction	10,020'	1.1	99.1	11S 334430E 4131717N
Rose Lake junction	10,030'	0.2	99.3	11S 334188E 4131442N
Marie Lake outlet	10,550'	1.4	100.7	11S 334212E 4129777N
Selden Pass	10,900'	1.0	101.7	11S 334059E 4128480N

here, you will find several sandy tent sites nestled among pines at the southeast end of the lake.

You then descend increasingly forested benches interspersed with openings surrounding granite slabs. Alongside a rock outcrop, clusters of bright, rose-pink flowers on the shrub rock spiraea are likely to catch your attention. Before long, you pass several campsites under open lodgepole cover and then ford Silver Pass Creek. The track soon skirts the southwestern edge of a large meadow with a meandering stream. In early summer, its edges are lined by western bistort, with tall stalks and dense heads of small white flowers. This species slowly disappears from the meadow community as you continue south. There is both a large stock camp and several smaller sites across the meadow, only easily accessed once water levels are low. As you round the next corner, the valley drops steeply in front of you and the vista opens up. Before you tackle the loose, rocky switchbacks, take a brief break to enjoy the waterfall and beautiful granite slabs to your left (east). Partway down the slope, the trail fords Silver Pass Creek again. This can be a dangerous crossing because of the dashing cascades above and below you. With luck, though, the well-placed boulders will be above the water and you can use them to carefully work your way across. Either way, shoes are best left on for this crossing. (You may read this description of gushing water and laugh, for this stretch of river can also run dry.) You drop steeply into the valley below, working your way down switchbacks while admiring spectacular slabs and superb junipers. Continued switchbacks bring you to a crossing of the North Fork of Mono Creek, another very dangerous ford under high flows, as the creek bed is rocky and the water turbulent, making footing difficult. (Having to make two such wretched crossings, one right after the other seems very unfair.) Immediately after the crossing, you reach the junction with the trail to Mott Lake [8,990' – 3.6/85.2] and a small campsite. The lush canyon leading to Mott Lake makes a lovely detour if you're in search of a wildflower walk.

Just beyond the junction, you enter lush Pocket Meadow, which, among other species, is filled with tall, yellow, sunflower-like flowers, Bigelow's sneezeweed. After a long meander at the meadow's edge, dry, rocky switchbacks resume; there is one campsite at the south end of the meadow and others in shelves along the descent. The presence of quaking aspens indicates areas subjected to disturbance, usually from avalanches. They are the first tree species to regrow following such disturbances, and they often even continue to grow after being flattened by recurring avalanches. The bright blue, tubular flowers of azure penstemon greet you as you descend. At times, the grade lessens and you reenter sections of mixed conifer forest and cross open slabs dotted with western junipers. After the junction with the Mono Creek Trail [8,350' – 1.4/86.6], you turn westward to travel alongside Mono Creek. (If you are in search of an unoccupied campsite, you will find several sites a short distance up the Mono Creek Trail, but be sure to collect water at the junction.) The grade briefly eases and you pass a larger campsite. The forest now consists of towering Jeffrey pines, occasional western junipers, and stands of white fir. After a few rocky switchbacks, you ford the North Fork of Mono Creek one last time. Once again, the water flow may be high and difficult, but at least here the river bottom is flat, broad, and covered with small pebbles (not boulders!); there are small campsites to either side of the crossing. The next junction you reach, at Quail Meadows, is with the Lake Edison Trail [7,900' – 1.4/88.0], which leads to the Lake Edison ferry landing and the Vermilion Valley Resort (VVR), a hospitable resupply stop for JMT and PCT travelers (see page 24 for resupply information, and Appendix A for lateral trail information). There is no camping

(Continued on page 122)

Which Way to VVR?

There is much discussion about how to get to and from the Vermillion Valley Resort, generally known as VVR. If you are coming from the north, most people leave the JMT at the Quail Meadows junction, and all the routes described in the table (see opposite page) assume that you do that. (If you are hiking northbound, the assumption is that you rejoin the JMT at this junction; just invert all the elevation gains and losses.) All the choices reconverge with the JMT by the Bear Creek junction, so distances and elevation gain on both lateral trails and the JMT are summed to that point. For each choice in the table, the mileage, elevation gain and loss, advantages and disadvantages are listed. You will immediately note that the elevation change is nearly identical for all options; you get to choose the method, but you do have to get across Bear Ridge—you choose between the JMT, the Bear Ridge Trail, or the Bear Creek cutoff. So instead of focusing on how much elevation you will gain or the minor differences in distance, contemplate what type of scenery you prefer and whether you mind missing part of the JMT.

Note that the map on pages 124–125 shows how these trails fit together.

(Continued from page 121)

at the junction, but you will find several choices along the JMT once you cross the bridge to the south. There are also campsites close to the ferry wharf if you're headed to VVR.

The JMT veers briefly east, to cross Mono Creek on a steel footbridge, and soon passes several campsites. Beyond is a charming meadow dotted with mounds of calcium carbonate deposited by springs. You then step across several small streams and seeps and begin the 2,000-foot climb up Bear Ridge. There may be no water for the next 5 miles up and over Bear Ridge, so it is advisable to fill your water bottles before beginning the ascent and be sure to start the climb with enough daylight to reach the shoulder's far side. Fortunately, the trail is well graded and mostly under partial forest cover, making the interminable switchbacks more tolerable.

About halfway up the climb, the trail sidles east toward a small, seasonal stream—a good place to dunk your head and cool off. At the base of the climb, western white pines, lodgepole pines, and a few western junipers dominate the tree cover, but with increasing elevation

ROUTE	TOTAL DISTANCE: QUAIL MDWS JCT » VVR » BEAR CREEK JCT	TOTAL ELEVATION: QUAIL MDWS JCT » VVR » BEAR CREEK JCT	ADVANTAGES	DISADVANTAGES
Edison ferry both directions and JMT over Bear Ridge to Bear Creek JCT	10.7 (3.0 off JMT + 6.7 on JMT)	+2,300, -1,200	• The entire length of the JMT • Beautiful view toward Selden Pass from the top of Bear Ridge • A well-graded, quiet, shady walk	• $19 RT for ferry • Ferry only runs twice a day (or +4.3 miles to walk one way)
Edison ferry and Bear Ridge Trail to JMT and JMT to Bear Creek JCT	8.5 (1.5 to ferry + 4.9 up Bear Ridge Trail + 2.1 on JMT)	+2,400, -1,300	• 2 miles shorter than other options • Much of the walk is shaded • Beautiful view toward Selden Pass from the top of Bear Ridge	• $12 for ferry + $10 for ride to TH • Ride to TH only twice a day (or add ~2 miles) • Not very scenic • +4.3 miles one way if ferry isn't running
Edison ferry and Bear Creek cutoff and Bear Creek Trail	10.8 (1.5 to ferry + 9.3 along the Bear Creek cutoff and Bear Creek trails)	+2,430, -1,330	• Truly beautiful walk • Follow a spectacular length of river for several miles	• $12 for ferry + $10 for ride to TH • Ride to TH only twice a day (or add ~2.5 miles) • Longest route—just barely • More of walk at lower, hotter elevations • +4.3 miles one way if ferry isn't running

and changing slope, you will pass through many different conifer communities. Next, white firs dominate the forest, giving way to a forest of western white pines, red firs, and mountain hemlocks as you continue up. Where the grade lessens, the forest is again a mix of lodgepole and western white pines, transitioning to pure lodgepole pine stands along the dry, flat, sandy top of Bear Ridge. Ground cover is variable but nearly always sparse, with bitter dogbane, rockcress, white-veined wintergreen, and alpine prickly currant all common. At the south end of Bear Ridge, you reach the junction with the Bear Ridge Trail, another alternative for reaching Lake Thomas Edison [9,870' – 4.6/92.6], and also the starting point for a detour to Volcanic Knob (see page 214). The south side of Bear Ridge could not be more different from the landscape you just passed through: It is well watered, with many seeps

(Continued on page 128)

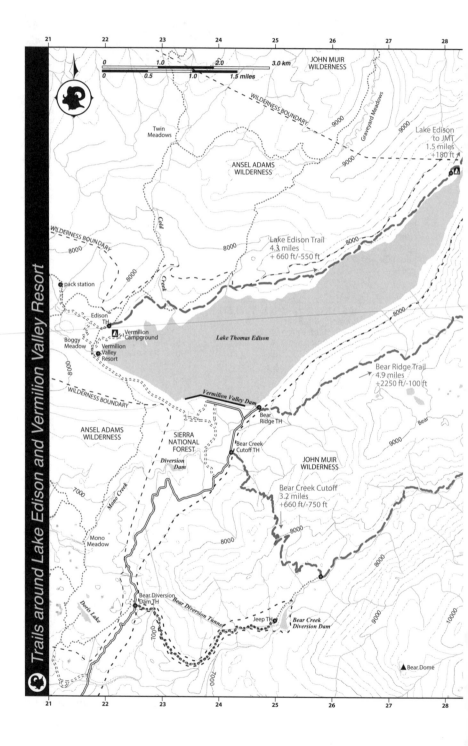

Trails around Lake Edison and Vermilion Valley Resort

JOHN MUIR
WILDERNESS

0   1.0   2.0   3.0 km
0   0.5   1.0   1.5 miles

WILDERNESS BOUNDARY

Twin
Meadows

ANSEL ADAMS
WILDERNESS

Cold Creek

WILDERNESS BOUNDARY

8000

pack station

Edison
TH

Vermilion
Campground

Boggy
Meadow

Vermilion
Valley
Resort

WILDERNESS BOUNDARY

Lake Thomas Edison

Graveyard Meadows

9000

9000

Lake Edison
to JMT
1.5 miles
+180 ft

Lake Edison Trail
4.3 miles
+ 660 ft/-550 ft

8000

8000

Bear Ridge Trail
4.9 miles
+2250 ft/-100 ft

Bear

Vermilion Valley Dam

Bear
Ridge TH

Bear Creek
Cutoff TH

ANSEL ADAMS
WILDERNESS

SIERRA
NATIONAL
FOREST

Diversion
Dam

JOHN MUIR
WILDERNESS

9000

Bear Creek Cutoff
3.2 miles
+660 ft/-750 ft

8000

8000

Mono Creek

7000

Mono
Meadow

8000

Bear Diversion
Dam TH

Bear Diversion Tunnel

7000

Jeep TH

Bear Creek
Diversion Dam

9000

10000

Dads Lake

7000

Bear Dome

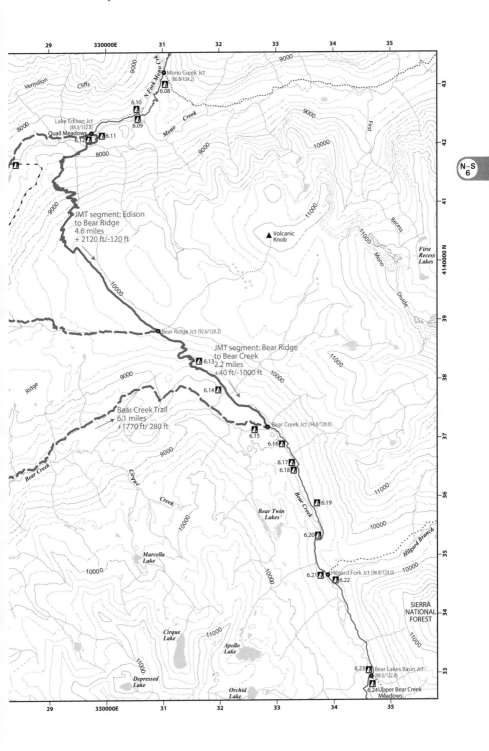

N–S 6

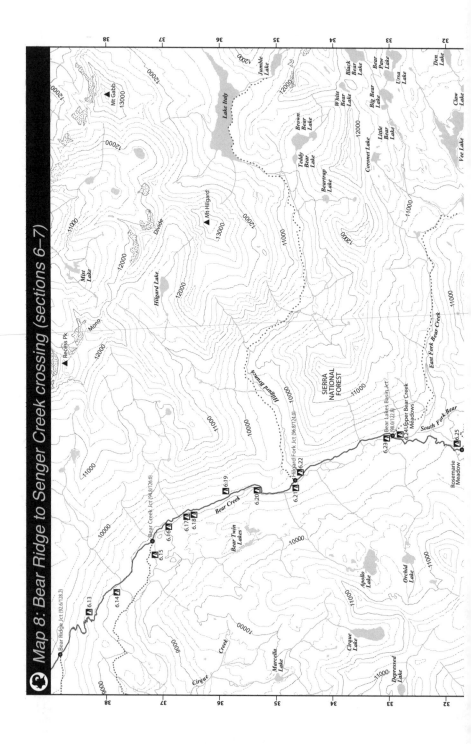

Map 8: Bear Ridge to Senger Creek crossing (sections 6–7)

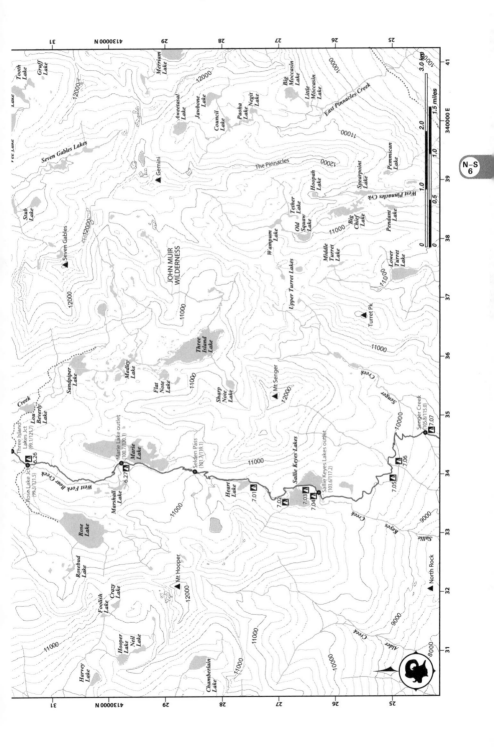

N-S
6

(Continued from page 123)

covered by wildflowers and dense vegetation. The dry, sandy benches in between are dotted with western junipers. From many points, you have a beautiful vista north to Seven Gables. Among the many flowers dotting the wet landscape, two tall ones are ranger's buttons, with tall heads that bear many small, white balls of flowers on branching stalks, and arrowleaf ragwort, with heads of small, straggly looking, yellow, daisylike flowers, and large leaves shaped like acute triangles. Both are common species at nearly every stream crossing in the montane and subalpine zones. Where the trail sidles close to an unmapped seasonal stream, you will encounter a large campsite beneath Jeffrey pines—a beautiful spot. When the grade lessens, you continue south across dry slopes, broken with outcrops of slab. In many stretches the ground is rocky and uneven—somewhat slowgoing as your stride is continually broken. The landscape slowly transitions to wetter forest with small stream crossings and muddy sections, and you shortly reach the Bear Creek Junction [8,940' – 2.2/94.8]. This track leads down spectacular Bear Creek to the Lake Thomas Edison area via the Bear Diversion Dam four-wheel-drive road, providing the shortest access to the post office at Mono Hot Springs, or the Bear Creek Cutoff, providing a fairly direct route to VVR (see page 24 and Appendix A for details).

Now in the beautiful canyon of rollicking Bear Creek and parallel-ing the creek on its east bank, the JMT begins a very gradual rise through lodgepole pine–dominated forest and passes numerous campsites. Bear Creek, in stretches lined by granite slabs, contains enticing swimming holes when the water is low, and impressive cascades when the water level is high. In places, the lodgepole forest gives way to openings with dry sedge meadows. Common in these meadows are mountain pretty-faces, Leichtlin's mariposa lily, and Parish's yampah. En route, you pass many campsites. You traipse along to the Hilgard Fork junction, an unmaintained trail that leads up to Lake Italy and then over Italy Pass [9,320' – 2.0/96.8]. Beyond is multistranded Hilgard Creek: The first two branches can be crossed on logs, but you will likely need to wade the third during high flow. There are campsites on either side of the cross-ings. Continuing through denser lodgepole forest, the JMT is farther from the river here and the vegetation is quite marshy, providing limited camping possibilities. Just as you exit the forest cover, there is one camp-site alongside slabs to the west of the trail. You quickly approach the junction with an unmaintained trail that leads up the East Fork of Bear Creek to the Bear Lakes Basin [9,580' – 1.3/98.0], and many campsites

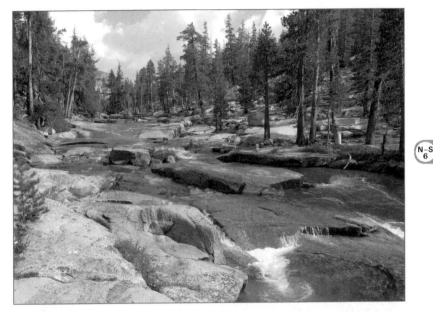

Bear Creek

along the eastern bank of Bear Creek. The JMT fords Bear Creek, often a difficult crossing in early summer, especially since the deep, swift water can combine with swarms of mosquitoes. However, by late season, flow decreases and the abundant western blueberry bushes lining the banks of the stream may yield an appetizing snack after you've hopped across the creek on rocks.

Beyond the crossing, the grade increases to a moderate climb through dry lodgepole forest, switchbacking upward to where the trail crosses the West Fork of Bear Creek, currently on a large log, to reach Rosemarie Meadow. After the crossing, look east (left) of the trail for campsites—there are many along the bluff here. Just after the final campsites, you meet a trail that departs east for Three Island Lake and Lou Beverly Lake [10,020' – 1.1/99.1]. Before long, the trail sidles out of the forest and into Rosemarie Meadow, providing good views of pyramid-shaped Mt. Hooper to the south. From the south end of the meadow, a trail climbs southwest to Rose Lake [10,030' – 0.2/99.3], a worthwhile 2-mile round-trip detour for a quiet afternoon or a secluded camp. Open, wet subalpine to alpine meadows, like this one, are good places to spot either spotted sandpipers or water pipits, two birds that occur sporadically throughout the Sierra on high-elevation, wet, hummocky meadows. Lemmon's paintbrush, mountain laurel, dwarf bilberry, and

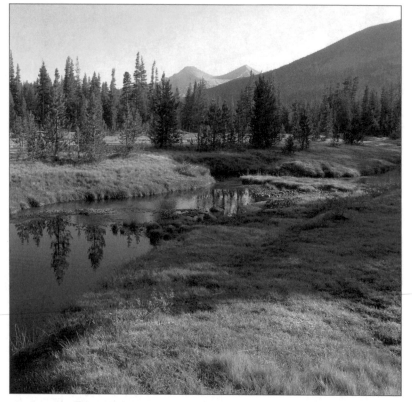

Rosemarie Meadow

Panorama north from Selden Pass

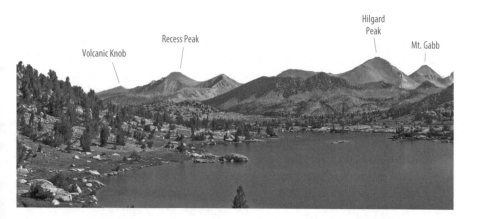

primrose monkeyflower are all common species here. There are camp-sites in the slabs just above Rosemarie Meadow and also just across the creek along the trail to Rose Lake.

The trail now climbs steadily, passing scattered mountain hemlocks and whitebark pines, as it approaches Marie Lake. En route, you also pass a few large glacial erratics, notable because dark-colored rock fragments are embedded in an otherwise light-colored granite. This rock, originally from a small outcrop just east of Mt. Hooper, was transported downslope by a glacier. Rounding a bend, you reach Marie Lake, a picturesque lake that fills a large, shallow basin trimmed and underlain by granite slabs, creating an oddly shaped lake dotted with islands. Several small campsites, often with open vistas northward, can be found on sandy patches near the outlet [10,550' – 1.3/100.7]. Skirting the lake's west shore, you begin the final climb to Selden Pass. You are slowly climbing into the alpine, and much like on the north side of Silver Pass, the sandy soil is scattered with small plants that you will notice only if you stare at your feet. Be sure to turn and look northward, as the views of Marie Lake, with the peaks crowning the Mono Recesses in the background, are more open before you reach the summit. You will undoubtedly take another breather atop the pass, an almost quaint gap between the light-colored granite walls and boulders [10,900' – 1.0/101.7].

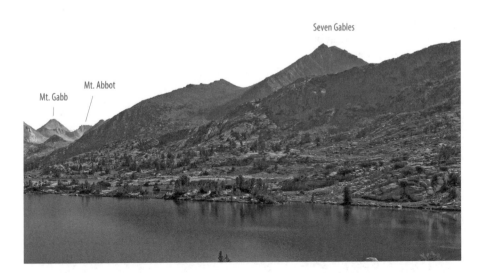

Seven Gables

Mt. Abbot

Mt. Gabb

SECTION 7.

Selden Pass to Muir Pass: South Fork of the San Joaquin River (27.4 miles)

Your final section within the San Joaquin drainage begins with a long downhill descent and ends with an even longer climb. It also marks a transition within your journey, as you pass the halfway point and then enter the ever-higher lake basins of the southern Sierra. As you begin your descent down rocky switchbacks, hunt for two related species, granite gilia and spreading phlox. Both have woody bases, needlelike leaves, and white, five-petaled, somewhat tubular flowers. Granite gilia is taller and spinier, with petals whose bases form a tight cone, while the petal tips are more open. In contrast, spreading phlox crawls along the ground and has petals whose ends stick out at right angles. Descending both sandy, dry slopes and wetter ones, along seeps or small patches of meadow, you pass little Heart Lake's east shore and cross its outlet, Sallie Keyes Creek, twice. A small party will find

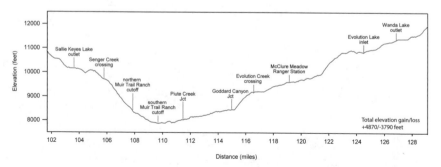

LOCATION	ELEVATION	DISTANCE FROM PREVIOUS POINT	CUMULATIVE DISTANCE	UTM COORDINATES
Selden Pass	10,900'	—	101.7	11S 334059E 4128480N
Sallie Keyes outlet crossing	10,180'	1.9	103.6	11S 333700E 4126292N
Senger Creek	9,740'	2.2	105.8	11S 334732E 4124433N
northern Muir Trail Ranch cutoff	8,410'	2.1	107.9	11S 334050E 4123185N
southern Muir Trail Ranch cutoff	7,900'	1.8	109.7	11S 334958E 4121342N
Piute Creek junction	8,050'	1.8	111.5	11S 337416E 4121220N
Goddard Canyon junction	8,480'	3.5	115.0	11S 340763E 4117572N
Evolution Creek wade	9,190'	1.6	116.6	11S 341942E 4117874N
McClure Meadow Ranger Station	9,630'	2.5	119.1	11S 345302E 4116963N
Evolution Lake inlet	10,860'	5.4	124.5	11S 349857E 4113827N
Wanda Lake outlet	11,380'	2.3	126.8	11S 349280E 4110505N
Muir Pass	11,980'	2.3	129.1	11S 351621E 4108409N

N–S
7

a campsite with open views near Heart Lake's outlet. The JMT continues downward and arrives at the Upper Sallie Keyes Lake; look along its northern shore for camping. The trail crosses Sallie Keyes Creek between the two lakes and follows the west shore of the lower lake. Along this stretch, there are many large campsites beneath lodgepole cover. A row of especially impressive lodgepole pines lines the bank of the lake; they are uncrowded and artistic, as if each were intentionally placed. At the outlet of the lower lake, you will cross Sallie Keyes Creek one final time on a logjam [10,180' – 1.9/103.6]. In case of an emergency, there is sometimes a ranger staying at the snow survey cabin 0.4 mile south of the lakes, located on the east side of the trail.

Below Sallie Keyes Lakes, the JMT curves southeast through a meadow and then into open lodgepole forest. A short distance onward, and just after a more open knob, are a couple of nice campsites. Water from a fork of Senger Creek is just a few steps farther down the trail. You cross the creek and proceed through a marshy meadow. More switchbacks, including a section passing large chinquapin-covered boulders, bring you to Senger Creek and some quite small campsites [9,740' – 2.2/105.8].

You now begin a long, dry drop into the river canyon far below. The grade is continuous, with no benches for camping. The open slope is mostly covered by large manzanita bushes and whitethorn, although a variety of other shrubs and herbs occasionally appear. Fox sparrows and green-tailed towhees enjoy this vegetation and may be seen hopping in and out of the bushes. The brown, slightly streaked sparrows are a bit larger than other sparrows that you may be familiar with, while the towhees have yellowish wings and a red cap; they are often sitting like sentinels atop branches, diving into the thickets once you approach. Look across the valley at some impressive avalanche chutes that have denuded the entire slope. Likely longing for shade, you will be appreciative as you slowly reenter tree cover, composed of mostly Jeffrey pines with scattered western junipers, and then reach a lateral to Florence Lake, the so-called northern cutoff [8,410' – 2.1/107.9]. It is thus known because this is the cutoff that southward-walking JMT hikers take to reach either the Muir Trail Ranch (MTR), a food drop depot, or Florence Lake (see Appendix A for further route description). Blayney Hot Springs is also accessed by this trail, but the public hot springs are on the southwestern side of the San Joaquin, and crossing the river to reach the hot springs can be dangerous, or impossible, during high flow.

The JMT, continuing in the direction signposted as KINGS CANYON, makes a gradual traversing descent to the South Fork of the San Joaquin River. Passing a small spring, the route is initially shaded while, lower down it, you cross both slopes of manzanita and whitethorn and stretches of open slab with Jeffrey pines and junipers, reaching the main branch of the Florence Lake Trail, or the southern cutoff, once on the valley floor [7,900' – 1.8/109.7]. If you have left the trail to pick up a food cache at MTR, and you do not mind missing a short stretch of the JMT, this is the junction where you will continue your southward journey on the JMT.

The JMT now diverges from the river, crossing over open, rocky, dry knobs of metamorphic rock with sedge meadows and scattered western junipers and Jeffrey pines. This open, flat valley of dark-colored rock is markedly different from anything you have seen to the north, or anything you will see to the south. Take your time to enjoy the majestic trees. Northern flickers, a species of woodpecker that feeds mostly on the ground, can be common at these elevations. They are easily identified by their red-orange underwings, which are visible in flight. Continuing along at the boundary between the forest river valley and the scrubby slope, your feet will feel the hard cobbles underfoot, especially noticeable if you have just picked up a heavy load of food. These are old flood deposits, left behind by massive flows that ripped down Piute Creek. Notice how rounded many of the rocks are and also how many different geologic origins they have, indicating they've been transported from many different sub-drainages. Continuing along, you reach a junction with the Piute Pass Trail, one branch of which goes north through Humphreys Basin and over Piute Pass to North Lake, while the other fork ascends French Canyon to Pine Creek Pass [8,050' – 1.8/111.5] (see Appendix A). The JMT, however, heads right, and as you cross turbulent Piute Creek on a steel footbridge, you leave behind John Muir Wilderness and enter Kings Canyon National Park. Nearby is a large, Jeffrey pine-shaded flat with numerous well-used and welcome campsites separated by chaparral thickets. Along the next stretch, there are often small sites on benches above the river.

N–S
7

Leaving Piute Creek behind, the JMT begins a gradual traverse across the dry, sunny southwest canyon wall. Often far below the trail, the green waters of the South Fork of the San Joaquin River roll and tumble over ledges of dark, metamorphic rock. A Townsend's solitaire may be perched atop one of the western junipers, flying above the stream in search of insects. This brown bird is identified by the yellow-beige pattern visible on its wings when it flies, as well as by its melodious song. Swarms of violet-green swallows also dive playfully above the water. By midsummer, rufous hummingbirds are likely sucking nectar from the abundant flowers. At night, bats emerge, likely from crevices in the steep metamorphic wall to the west, to feed on insects. Rounding a corner you pass a rock inscribed with MUIR TRAIL 1917, likely commemorating the construction of a new bridge across Piute Creek as funding for the JMT first became available. As you approach Aspen Meadow, you leave the open slopes behind. Moreover, the "meadow" is now a forest, a mixture of quaking aspen, lodgepole pine, white fir, and the occasional western juniper; it too has suffered from a recent blowdown. You continue upstream, soon back in the open, taking in the impressive canyon walls and the turbulent waters that flow over the fractured rock. Common species on this dry slope include western eupatorium, a late-blooming species with a collection of light lavender heads, and many I have previously described, including granite gilia, scarlet penstemon, and ocean spray.

(Continued on page 139)

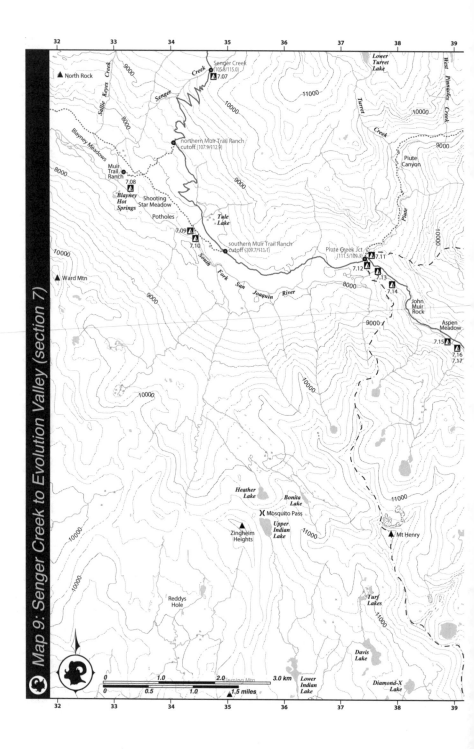

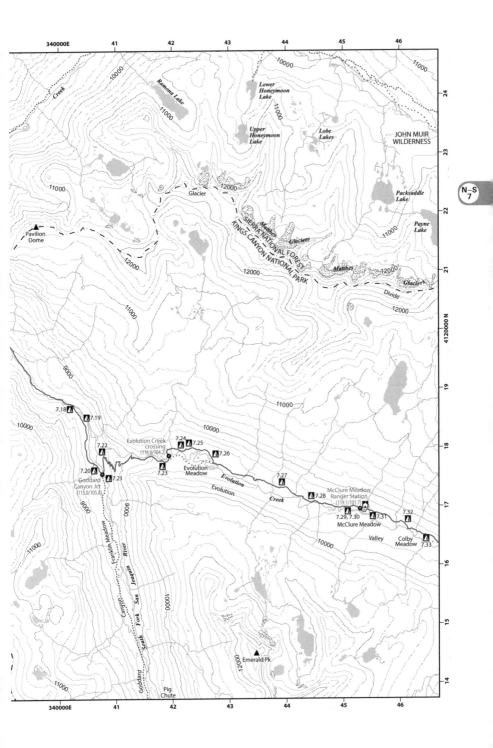

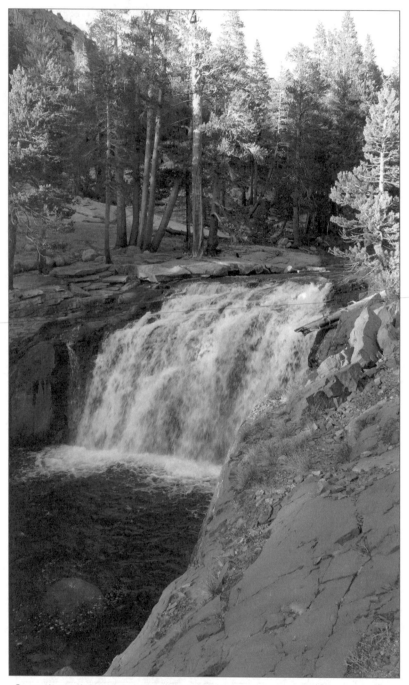

Cascade on the ascent to Evolution Valley

(Continued from page 135)

At the end of a long, flat traverse, you cross the river on a footbridge, pass a use trail to some campsites just northwest of the bridge, and continue upstream, now in lodgepole forest. The trail curves south, passing through drier and then wetter stretches of lodgepole forest as you head upstream. Kelley's tiger lilies grow alongside a small creek. After an easy but possibly shoes-off creek crossing, you reach a junction where the Goddard Canyon/Hell For Sure Pass Trail continue south up the river, while the JMT turns east, crossing the South Fork of the San Joaquin on a log footbridge [8,480' – 3.5/115.0].

Just over the bridge, the JMT hooks briefly north past some campsites before tackling east-trending switchbacks that take you up the canyon's steep east wall into one of the Sierra's most exquisite regions, Evolution Valley and Evolution Basin. Take a breather as you climb past stately junipers, enjoy the panoramic vista, and especially look across to the west canyon wall. Note the streams and waterfalls flowing down deeply incised and nearly straight fractures in the metamorphic rock; granite rarely forms such straight, narrow channels down a cliff face. This black rock comprises the Goddard pendant, one of the largest masses of metavolcanic rock in the Sierra. Similar to the rocks in the Ritter Range, this is material that erupted between 160 and 130 million years ago as subduction was occurring along the edge of the North American plate and the Ancestral Sierra was a chain of volcanoes. Continued tectonic action around 90 million years ago formed the granitic plutons in the area, and simultaneously displaced and metamorphosed the volcanic rocks into what you see today. Outcrops of the Goddard pendant were first visible as you descended to the South Fork of the San Joaquin and you will continue seeing the dark rock across Muir Pass and down to Grouse Meadow.

As the slope eases, the bedrock you are walking on again becomes granite, and Evolution Creek, to your north, changes character. Suddenly, you are walking alongside foaming cascades and deep, rounded holes, quite different from the steep-walled gorges a few miles back. A lateral trail heads south to a collection of campsites high on a bench and, presently, the JMT reaches a creek crossing [9,190' – 1.6/116.6]. This is the main crossing of Evolution Creek and the one that should be used when water levels are low. However, if the flow is dangerous, continue on the use trail up the southern bank of the creek to a second crossing; it is similarly deep, but there you will be in Evolution Meadow, without dangerous rapids just downstream.

As you continue upstream, around the northern edge of Evolution Meadow, you will pass several campsites occupying open areas beneath lodgepole cover. Along the trail, the forest floor is dry, except in areas with small seeps. Here, heath vegetation dominates and arnicas are a typical sight. Along small trickles, the swamp onion, with a tall stalk, purple flowers, and a pungent onion smell, is a common plant. Beyond Evolution Meadow is a stretch of forest that opens up as you reach McClure Meadow. A summer ranger is stationed on the slopes just north of the meadow, but the path to the cabin is easily missed if you are walking east [9,630' – 2.6/119.1]. The campsites fringing McClure Meadow are justifiably popular for the views they offer—to the west lies a steep monolith, the Hermit, while along the eastern skyline are the first of the Evolution Basin peaks—Mt. Mendel, Mt. Darwin, Mt. Spencer, and Mt. Huxley. The Hermit is an arête; its steep front marks where two glaciers once merged together, that pouring from McGee Canyon (directly to the south) and the one descending from Evolution Basin (farther southeast). The Hermit was therefore simultaneously carved from two sides, producing the striking landform. Arêtes are most obvious when walking up-canyon; the peaks might be quite rounded and unspectacular when viewed from behind.

If you look at the elevation profile for this section (on page 132), you will note that the distance from the low point, at the southern JMT cutoff, to the top of Muir Pass is divided into approximately three sections. First is the long, gradual climb up the South Fork of the San Joaquin, truncated by the abrupt climb as you leave Goddard Canyon for the hanging Evolution Valley. The many miles up Evolution Valley are again gentle, but you now leave Evolution Valley and climb steeply up into another hanging valley, in which Evolution Basin and its famous lakes are found. A hanging valley forms when the glacier in the side valley cannot erode its valley floor as quickly as does the larger glacier in the main valley, creating a steep drop-off. At the first step, Goddard Canyon was eroded more quickly than Evolution Valley, and at the second, the drainage to the McGee Lakes was more eroded than Evolution Basin.

Continuing your gradual ascent and crossing several tributaries, you reach Colby Meadow and more campsites. Your route is still largely within dry lodgepole forest, with occasional excursions to the edge of meadows or onto granite slabs. This leads to the ford the multibranched stream that drains Darwin Canyon; while not difficult, it is potentially cumbersome. Pass a small campsite on an open slab, and begin the climb to Evolution Basin. For the next 10 miles, the only camping options are above treeline and in locations suited for just one or two tents, so if it is getting late in the day, consider stopping below this climb, and give yourself a full day to enjoy Evolution Basin.

Just at the top of the last switchback is the unsigned junction with a use trail to spectacular Darwin Bench, well worth a detour to camp or to eat lunch. Alternatively, you may travel up over Lamarck Col, a popular cross-country route. As the gradient lessens, the forest thins, the views open up, and you find yourself walking on sand patches between granite slabs and rocky outcrops. Such habitat is ideal for the white-tailed ptarmigan, an introduced species whose population remarkably stabilized at relatively low numbers.

Within a short distance, you leave the last stunted trees behind, reach the outlet of Evolution Lake, find a few small campsites north of the lake's outlet, and look forward to your 5-mile tromp through undeniably spectacular Evolution Basin. Make sure you have many hours to wander upward and to sit and stare. This basin is also steeped in JMT history: in July 1895 Theodore Solomons, the visionary of the JMT, named the first six peaks of the Evolution Range after the most prominent figures in the new field of evolutionary biology: Darwin, Fiske, Haeckel, Huxley, Spencer, and Wallace, along with Evolution Lake. Although Solomons had first alighted on the idea of the JMT a decade earlier, it was on trips in 1895 and 1896 that he fleshed out his idea, in part while soaking up the landscape of Evolution Basin. During these summers, he traveled along the current JMT route as far as Muir Pass, but his parties then descended to the Middle Fork of the Kings by other routes. Their goal was to find a route between Yosemite and the South Fork of the Kings that stayed close to the crest and was passable by stock. Both years, then unnamed Muir Pass was buried beneath an enormous snowbank, and they searched farther west for alternatives. Finally, in 1907, a U.S. Geological Survey party crossed Muir Pass, and the following year, Joseph N. Le Conte used the pass as he continued scouting a route for the eventual JMT.

You skirt around the eastern shore of Evolution Lake, on a route constructed in the early 1990s to avoid the lake's sensitive shoreline; please stay away from the shore here. You are passing by the massive wall of scalloped ridges and gullies descending from Mt. Mendel, a later-named addition to the Evolution Peaks. Looping around, you reach Evolution Lake's inlet, crossed on a series of large granite blocks [10,860' – 5.4/124.5]. You continue up a gentle slope, passing sandy stretches dotted with small alpine plants, meadows dotted with a more

(Continued on page 144)

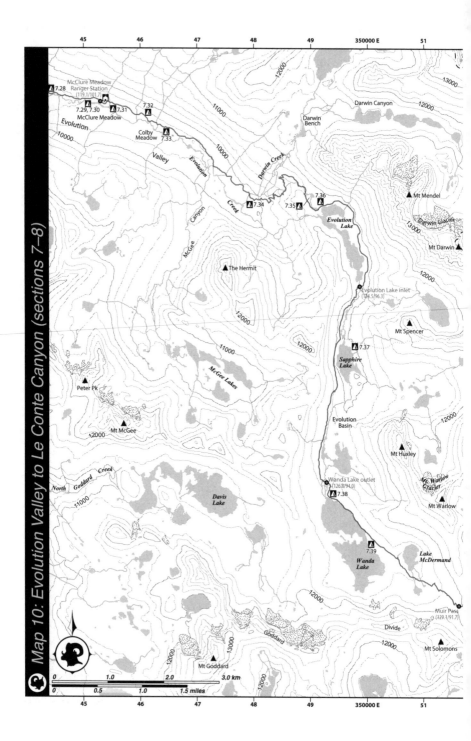

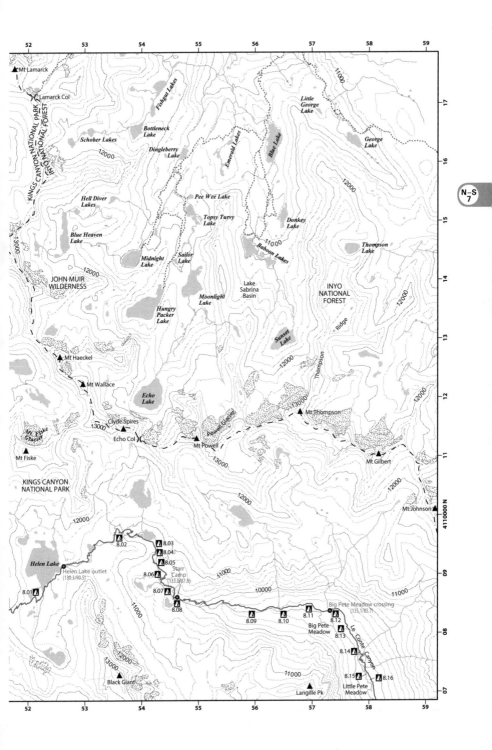

(Continued from page 141)

colorful selection of flowers, and to the east, a series of small lakes. The sandy flats often contain Muir's ivesia, one of the few plants to bear the name of this famous naturalist. These are small yellow flowers on long stalks with dense stalks of minute, fuzzy leaves that resemble a mouse's tail. Often growing together with frosted wild buckwheat, Muir's ivesia is a species that grows only in coarse sandy soils. In these same stretches, you may see the dwarf alpine paintbrush, not as dazzling and bright as the other species, but still elegantly colored. Growing just a few inches off the ground, the characteristic tubular flowers range from green to white to light pink, and the upper leaves sport a dainty white or pink edge. Meanwhile, Lemmon's paintbrush, with its magenta flowers, grows in the wetter meadows you pass. This is also the habitat of gray-crowned rosy finches, delightful little birds. They are common at high elevations, traveling in small groups and feeding on the insects that emerge from the alpine tarns or scavenging them from snowbanks.

As you make this climb, stop and admire the many glacial features that surround you. During the Pleistocene's glacial periods, Evolution Basin was scoured clean, and the polished granite, chatter marks, and abundant glacial erratics scattered across the landscape attest to the glaciers' presence. Chatter marks are the regular pattern of curved lines visible in the polished granite. They formed when a rock was scraped across the bedrock by the moving glacier. Since then, little soil formation has occurred, and the smooth granite slabs still dominate the landscape. Meanwhile, the upper sections of the highest peaks, Mt. Darwin and Mt. Mendel, were untouched by glaciers. Mt. Darwin's summit region is a broad plateau, the remnant of a gentle Sierra landscape that existed before a combination of uplift and river erosion, fine-tuned by glacial activity, created today's landforms. Take note of the chutes and ribs that decorate their western faces—these are avalanche chutes, whose exact locations are determined by the location of joints within the granite. The rock in the joints is more easily fractured and displaced by freeze-thaw activity, and the loose rock is then carried downslope by the snow. In many places in the Sierra, these avalanches not only remove rock, but also polish the chutes. Note that these giant slides are often truncated some distance above today's valley floor. The boundary between steep chute and nearly vertical wall marks the height to which the valley was once filled with ice and is called the trimline.

Near the outlet of stunning Sapphire Lake, the trail begins to climb up the west side of the valley, away from the drainage. If you were to leave the JMT here and head around the eastern shore of Sapphire

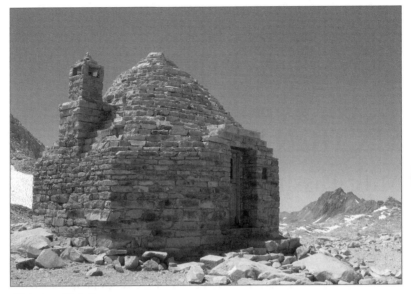

N–S
7

Hut atop Muir Pass

Lake, you would find a few small campsites in sandy patches along
the eastern shore of the lake. This is also the place to leave the trail if
you wish to climb Mt. Spencer, another arête, which is characteristically
steep when approached from the north, but has an easy ascent from the
southwest (see page 214). The grade eases again as you approach a pair
of unnamed lakes.

You now cross the multibranched outlet [11,380' – 2.3/126.8]
of Wanda Lake and soon reach the large lake, named for one of John
Muir's daughters. The views here are vast and impressively stark: the
light-colored granite, the intense blue of Wanda's waters, and the massive, dark pyramid of Mt. Goddard, the tallest of the peaks in the Goddard pendant.

Your trail follows Wanda's grassy east shore and climbs up the
gentle slope leading past Lake McDermand, finally ending at Muir Pass
[11,980' – 2.3/129.1]. Atop is a stone hut, built in 1930 and recently ren-
ovated, that is intended to provide emergency shelter during storms;
camping in it is, however, prohibited. George Frederick Schwarz, an
early Sierra Club supporter, provided the $5,810.48 to build it; much
like today, transporting materials to remote locations was expensive
and more than half the money went to pay for pack stock and packers.
And since a marmot is always on guard at the hut, don't let yourself
become too distracted reading this paragraph—keep your eyes on your
food at all times!

SECTION 8.

Muir Pass to Mather Pass: Middle Fork of the Kings River (22.0 miles)

A s you cross Muir Pass, you enter the Kings River drainage. With the exception of the 5 miles in the Rush Creek drainage, all the land you have traversed thus far drains into the San Francisco Bay. From here south, water reaches the ocean only in wet years — mind-boggling when you consider the vast quantities of snow that bury this country each winter! The water from the Kings and Kern drainages once flowed into Tulare Lake in the southern San Joaquin Valley, a vast wetland, but today *all* of the water is diverted for irrigation, and the Tulare lake bed is mostly agricultural land.

Vindicating Solomons for overlooking the relatively straightforward Muir Pass, snow does often linger on the east side of Muir Pass well into the summer, and you descend toward Helen Lake on either

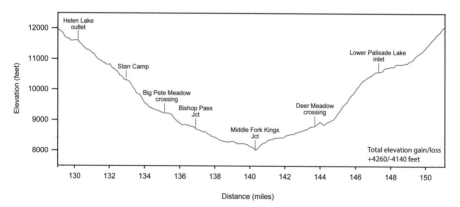

LOCATION	ELEVATION	DISTANCE FROM PREVIOUS POINT	CUMULATIVE DISTANCE	UTM COORDINATES
Muir Pass	11,980'	—	129.1	11S 351621E 4108409N
Helen Lake outlet	11,630'	1.2	130.3	11S 352635E 4109144N
Starr Camp	10,320	2.7	133.0	11S 354628E 4108611N
Big Pete Meadow creek crossing	9,240'	2.1	135.1	11S 357317E 4108373N
Bishop Pass junction	8,740'	1.8	136.9	11S 358394E 4106307N
Middle Fork junction	8,030'	3.4	140.3	11S 359641E 4101704N
Deer Meadow creek crossing	8,830'	3.4	143.7	11S 364332E 4101910N
Lower Palisade Lake outlet	10,600'	3.6	147.3	11S 367700E 4102388N
Mather Pass	12,100'	3.8	151.1	11S 370213E 4099138N

N–S
8

rocky-sandy switchbacks or across a well-trodden path in the snow. To the southeast lies the Black Giant, the northern end of the metamorphic Black Divide and an easy peak with an excellent vista if you have half a day to spare (see page 215). As you encircle Helen Lake, named for John Muir's other daughter, enjoy its brilliant blue waters and the surrounding colorful glaciated slabs. The trail passes near the contact between metamorphic and granitic rocks, passing a few small campsites and then crossing Helen Lake's outlet on boulders [11,630' – 1.2/130.3]. You follow the infant Middle Fork of the Kings River down an enticing little gorge, paved with dark rock. For stretches, the creek flows over the trail, but it is usually too small to impede your progress. Flowers appreciate the abundant moisture and color the base of steep walls. One species is the larger mountain monkeyflower, similar in shape to the primrose monkeyflower but much larger and growing in seeps, rather than meadows. The rocks here are dark, some decorated with colorful streaks of minerals; here you are in the contact zone between the granite and the rock of the Goddard pendant. Beyond, you reach a small, unnamed lake and follow the trail across the inlet stream, where the water spreads out into a meadow filled with dense patches of mountaineer shooting stars interspersed with cobble-paved waterways.

You continue downstream, at first past knobs of metamorphic rock, then cross back into granite, and shortly view your first stunted

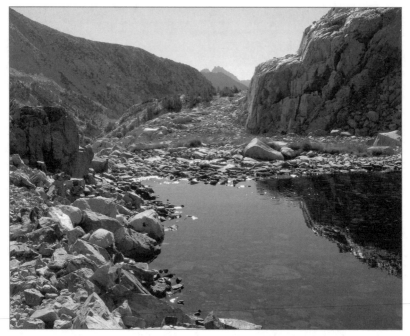

The headwaters of the Middle Fork of the Kings River

whitebark pine since Evolution Lake. Take note that granitic knobs are much more likely than metamorphic ones to contain small, flat, sandy patches that suffice as small campsites, since the granite often remains as unbroken slab, while the metamorphic rock decomposes into piles of boulders. Just above the 10,800-foot mark, you ford another series

Panorama east from Muir Pass

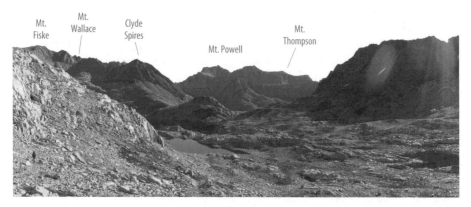

of inlet streams and encircle another unnamed lake; glimpse at its shores to see if a few mountain yellow-legged frogs are still able to live here. Good campsites with stunning views lie among the stunted trees on the knob to the east of its outlet. The JMT continues downward, switchbacking down a steeper slope, crossing the creek several times and passing small campsites to the east of the trail. Trickles of water abound, and the vegetation is lush. Clark's nutcrackers will be hopping among the treetops. Gaze up at the looming east face of the Black Giant and note how the peak's character changes at the contact between metamorphic and granitic rocks. Lower down, a few large campsites present themselves under open stands of tall lodgepole pines. You pass a large, marshy meadow and then a flat of young lodgepole pines, long ago named Starrs Camp. If you leave the trail here, you find abundant camping opportunities in the direction of the creek, positioned at the top of the steep drop into Le Conte Canyon [10,320' – 2.8/133.0]. This is also a good spot for a break; drop your backpack and walk to the creek's edge to *carefully* look at the cascading water and visit the banks of a small lake.

N–S
8

The stream now plunges downward and the trail switchbacks a bit more gradually down the north canyon wall through patchy forest. In wet sections, you will see large ferns and fireweed, which have clusters of quite large, four-petaled pink flowers on very tall stalks. Drier sections are dominated by shrubs, including manzanita and chinquapin. To navigate through one section, the trail had to be blasted out of the canyon's sheer granite wall, and when you read Joseph N. Le Conte's account

(Continued on page 152)

Black Giant

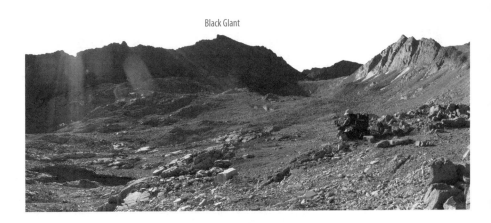

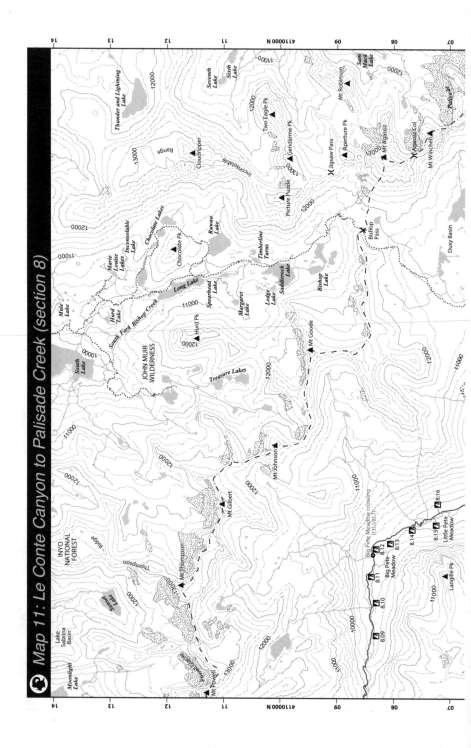

Map 11: Le Conte Canyon to Palisade Creek (section 8)

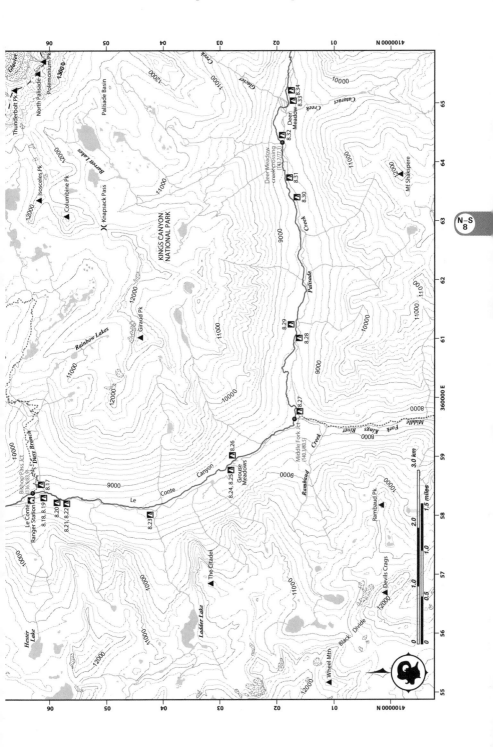

(Continued from page 149)

of crisscrossing the valley multiple times to navigate around the cliffs, you'll be glad for the work of the dynamite. The trail becomes ever rockier underfoot as you pound down increasingly dry slopes toward the valley bottom. Suddenly, the trail intersects the stream course, you reenter the forest, and come upon more campsites. Although there are stands of mountain hemlocks on steep, north-facing slopes, the river-bottom forest is dominated by lodgepole pines. You walk along the refreshingly soft trail through the forest, shortly crossing, on logs, the multibranched side stream that intersects the trail just before Big Pete Meadow [9,240' – 2.1/135.1]. Just after the crossing, you pass several small campsites and, farther along, a spur trail that leads to larger campsites along the main stream. For a short stretch, you emerge from the lodgepole forest onto a sandy slope with western junipers and phenomenal views westward to the steep face of Langille Peak. There is one small campsite here. You next come to Little Pete Meadow, which is, contrary to its name, large. The river meanders through here, and oxbow lakes that formed when the stream changed its course are visible. To the edge are dense stands of corn lilies: In spring, these look like ears of corn, but by summer they are taller and straggly. A few of these plants will have many-branched heads of white flowers, but most die back without flowering. There are a few campsites along the meadow's perimeter, including a large stock camp. Soon thereafter, the JMT reaches a junction with the Bishop Pass Trail [8,740' – 1.8/136.9], leading up into Dusy Basin and over Bishop Pass, the easiest route to the town of Bishop. From this same point, a spur trail heads west to the Le Conte ranger cabin.

Along the stretch of trail from here to the confluence of the Middle Fork of the Kings River and Palisade Creek, there are few campsites that are 100 feet from the trail and/or water. Remember that the Kings Canyon regulations allow you to camp in established campsites that are 25 feet from trail/water. You immediately pass a few campsites and then cross the turbulent Dusy Branch on a footbridge. The views along the entire length of Le Conte Canyon are beautiful, as you pass first Langille Peak and then approach the Citadel; both are steep, imposing summits. For stretches you are walking through dry, predominately lodgepole forest; for others, you head across dry, open slopes, often where avalanches or rockslides prevent a conifer forest from establishing. Slopes covered by downslope-oriented tree trunks and vegetated by scrubby aspens are indicative of avalanche activity. In these open sections, note a mixture of two different manzanitas. One, pinemat

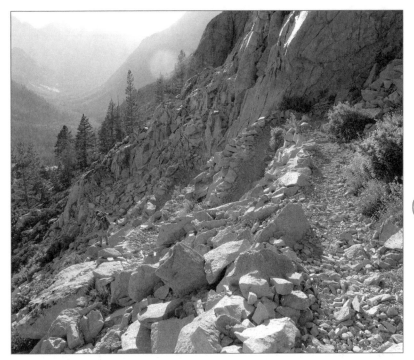

Ascending the Golden Staircase to the Palisade Lakes

manzanita, creeps along the ground, often under scattered tree cover, while the other, greenleaf manzanita, grows as a taller bush and has sticky glands on its leaf stalks. Both have scaly red bark, characteristic of all manzanita species. A few miles downstream, the trail passes Grouse Meadow, a long, skinny meadow with outstanding views of Le Conte Canyon and one of the largest blueberry patches in the Sierra—at least in late August of "good" years. You will find several campsites along its length. You continue downstream to the Middle Fork Trail junction [8,030' – 3.4/140.3], your lowest point until after the summit of Mt. Whitney. Several campsites are present here beneath tall Jeffrey pines. In the past, you could cross Palisade Creek on a bridge, but a flood has washed out all but the foundation, visible a short distance upstream, and the trail down the Middle Fork of the Kings is now difficult to access if water is high. To continue your history lesson: Until the switchbacks up the Golden Staircase, 3 miles ahead, were completed, hikers continued descending the Middle Fork of the Kings and

(Continued on page 156)

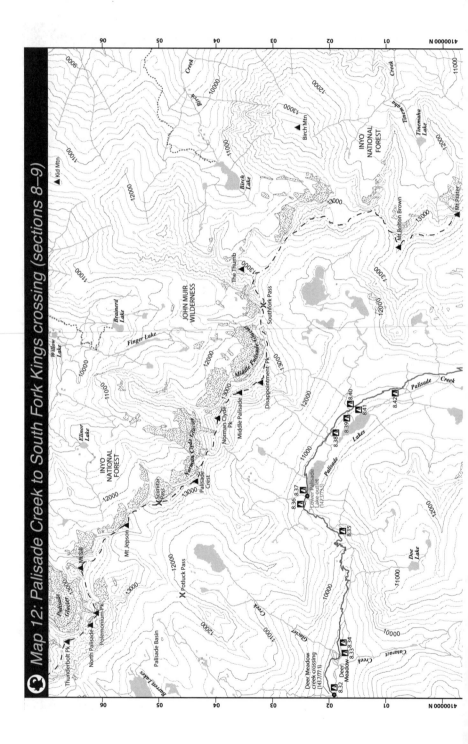

Map 12: Palisade Creek to South Fork Kings crossing (sections 8–9)

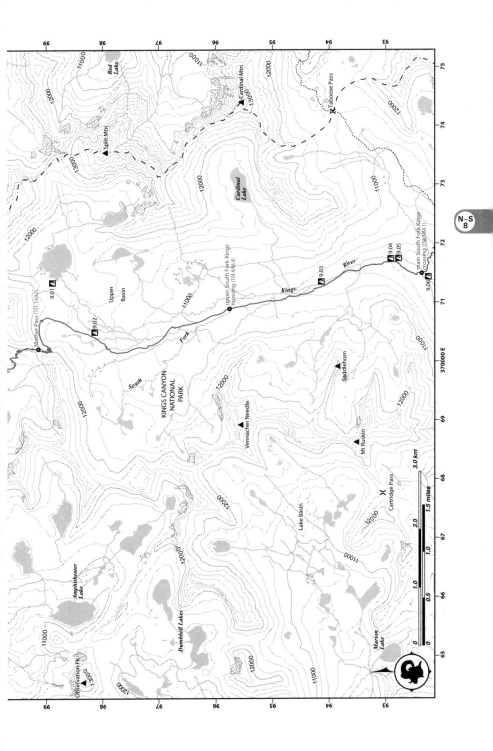

(Continued from page 153)

then ascended Cartridge Creek, some miles west, crossed Lake Basin, summited Cartridge Pass, and dropped down to the South Fork of the Kings, the river on the south side of Mather Pass. Most of these trails are now unmaintained and difficult to follow.

The JMT now turns eastward and, paralleling Palisade Creek, begins its long climb to Mather Pass. The next many miles have few campsites. Much of the next 3 miles was affected by the 2002 lightning-started Palisade Fire, and the landscape is dotted with charred tree trunks. Other sections are affected by regular avalanche activity and are overgrown with aspen scrub. In many places, the vegetation is lush and diverse, making for colorful flower displays in early summer. As the vegetation changes during the next many years, the location of campsites will change, but the best opportunities are undisturbed stands of trees near the river.

Just before Deer Meadow, you reenter undisturbed lodgepole forest and cross the stream draining Palisade Basin high above [8,830' – 3.4/143.7]. Heading south from the trail, you find a large area of shaded

Panorama north from Mather Pass

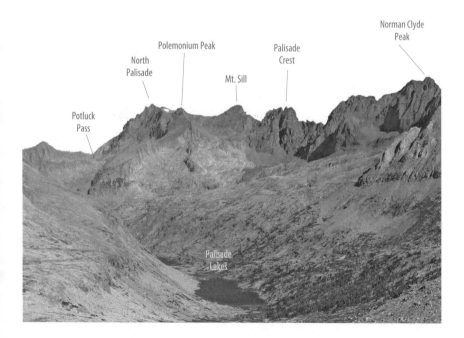

campsites in Deer Meadow, a lodgepole forest. An often-marshy section of trail then crosses many forks of Glacier Creek, draining another basin at the foot of the 14,000-foot northern Palisade Peaks, and enters another section of dense lodgepole forest with several camping opportunities.

Beyond, you exit forest cover and begin an exposed 1,500-foot climb up switchbacks known as the Golden Staircase. Impressively built walls form the foundation for the switchbacks that make for a steep climb up a much steeper headwall. Completed in 1938, this was the last section of the JMT to be constructed, and one of only two sections of the route that Le Conte was unable to navigate with stock on his 1908 expedition. For stretches, the trail is dry and rocky, while elsewhere, small seeps provide water and host a different community of plants. The drier sections are dominated by the evermore familiar wavyleaf paintbrush, scarlet penstemon, pennyroyal, and western eupatorium. Thickets of chinquapin grow alongside rocks. The wetter sections boast orange sneezeweed, swamp onion, Kelley's tiger lily, and great red paintbrush. Two other species in the wetter sites are the Sierra bog orchid, bearing very small, white, orchid-shaped flowers on leafy

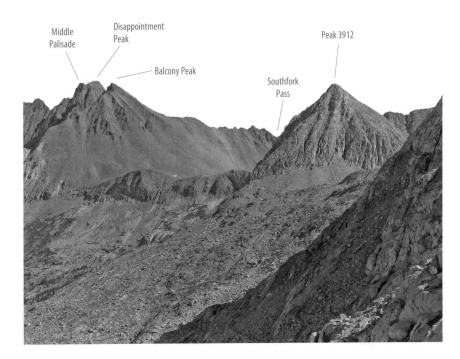

Middle Palisade Disappointment Peak Balcony Peak Southfork Pass Peak 3912

stalks, and alpine goldenrod, with short, yellow, ray petals that are dwarfed by the more sizable orange-yellow discs. As you climb higher, look along rocky walls for a pink-flowered shrub whose base emerges from cracks and whose stems literally hug the rock: rosy-petaled cliff-bush. The route-finding required to build this trail is impressive; notice how tight switchbacks take you up one gully, only to have it dead-end in cliffs. You next traverse seamlessly to the next passable gully, slowly working your way up the steep face. But also take breaks to look to tumbling Palisade Creek, which flows steeply down to Deer Meadow and on toward Devils Crags, the dark, jagged mass of pinnacles at the southern end of the Black Divide. The grade eases and you enjoy your final unbroken views down-canyon. For the final stretch to Palisade Lake, you pass small patches of meadow and climb next to short bluffs; you pass several small campsites as you ascend. You also pass the final mountain hemlocks on your southward journey. After fording a couple of tributaries, you reach the west end of the Lower Palisade Lake and enjoy your first broken view of the 14,000-foot Palisades [10,600' – 3.6/147.3]. On slabs to the north of the trail are a large collection of tent sites, sandy and barren, but what surroundings!

The trail bends southeastward, as it skirts the northeastern shores of the Palisade Lakes. You will see the steep granite walls to the south, the sharp-toothed Middle Palisade group to the north, and Mather Pass to the southeast. You ford an occasional stream, some of which may require a brief wade in early summer, and while traversing high above the Upper Palisade Lake, pass several view-rich campsites on small shelves among stunted whitebark pines. Once past the lakes, the trail turns south, traverses small meadows and soon begins the final ascent to the pass: switchbacks through amazingly barren talus. Only a few species can grow here; among them is the bright pink Sierra prim-rose. It is a southern Sierra species that is quite rare farther north in the Sierra. Within the cracks of granite slabs emerge clumps of stalks tufted by yellow flowers. These are dwarf ivesia, which are widespread and become one of the dominant species at the highest elevations, always emerging from such cracks. Finally, you reach Mather Pass—named for Stephen Mather, the first head of the National Park Service and a con-servation luminary who was much admired by his contemporaries—and enjoy a much-deserved break on the summit [12,100' – 3.8/151.1]. Looking at the awe-inspiring view to the north, you see the full length of the North and Middle Palisade peaks: Within view are six points that extend above the 14,000-foot mark.

SECTION 9.

Mather Pass to Pinchot Pass: South Fork of the Kings River (9.9 miles)

The view south from Mather Pass is equally fantastic: To the east is Split Mountain, the southernmost of the Palisade-area fourteeners. If you wish to take a layover day in the vicinity, it is a straightforward, if long, climb (see page 216). Due south is another of the JMT's spectacular alpine basins, lake-dotted Upper Basin, the headwaters of the South Fork of the Kings River. You descend moderately, first switch-backing down a sandy, bouldery slope, then curving east and beyond, resuming a southward bearing as you enter Upper Basin. Although no established campsites are visible from the trail, you can easily wander toward any of the tarns and may pitch your tent on flat, sandy, unvegetated patches. The scale of these tarns is so different from Evolution Basin's deep, giant lakes, but they are equally enticing. You can easily sit along their banks, sometimes on nearly bare sand, other times on

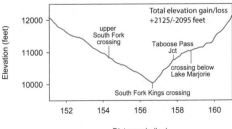

LOCATION	ELEVATION	DISTANCE FROM PREVIOUS POINT	CUMULATIVE DISTANCE	UTM COORDINATES
Mather Pass	12,100'	—	151.1	11S 370213E 4099138N
South Fork Kings crossing at the base of Upper Basin	10,830'	3.3	154.4	11S 370891E 4095758N
main South Fork Kings crossing	10,040'	2.3	156.7	11S 371500E 4092362N
Taboose Pass junction	10,760'	1.1	157.8	11S 371999E 4091444N
crossing below Marjorie Lake	11,050'	1.0	158.8	11S 372485E 4090166N
Pinchot Pass	12,130'	2.2	161.0	11S 374287E 4088510N

polished slabs, and stare at the collection of insects and perhaps small Pacific tree frog tadpoles racing about.

Beyond the tarns, you find yourself elevated from the surrounding landscape on a shallow, sandy ridge, the perfect habitat for frosted wild buckwheat, dwarf alpine paintbrush, and Muir's ivesia. This ridge is a moraine, a pile of boulders and sand deposited as the Tioga glaciers retreated 14,000 years ago. At its end, you drop back to the wetter landscape, crossing a few small tributaries en route. The gentle grade makes for easy going—all the better to appreciate the landscape. To the west are steep, glaciated, lighter-colored granite peaks, and to the east, darker, craggier, fractured ones, representing two different plutons from different eras and with different chemical compositions. The western peaks are made of the younger Cartridge Pass granodiorite,

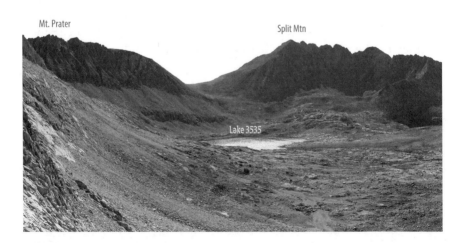
Mt. Prater   Split Mtn

Lake 3535

while Split Mountain is composed of the older Tinemaha granodiorite. In addition, stripes of colorful metamorphic rock outcrop just east of the Sierra crest here, but you will see them once near Pinchot Pass. Before any of the granites began to form, these metamorphic rocks were seafloor sediments, mostly deep sea mud, but interspersed with small calcium-carbonate reefs. As magma began pushing up against these sediments about 165 million years ago, they were heated, compressed, and twisted into the rocks we see today, while plutons formed beneath them. Much of the metamorphic rock has been eroded away, but stripes of it are still seen atop and embedded in the oldest of the granitic rocks. Along the JMT, you can see this contact zone from here south to Glen Pass. Just north of Taboose Pass, and barely visible from the JMT is Cardinal Mountain, a massive red peak with a white tip, sticks out to the southeast: The red material was once silt, while the white is marble, the remains of ocean critters deposited in a shallow reef environment. The first granitic rocks were also heated and deformed as they bashed against the preexisting sedimentary rocks, which is why they are so much more deformed and fractured than the beautiful massive granite to your west. As for the darker color, that is because the older granites have more iron and magnesium-bearing minerals than do the granites that formed later—see pages 58–59 for more information.

Forest cover increases as you descend and ford the South Fork of the Kings [10,830' – 3.3/154.4]. Over the next mile, snooping eastward, in the direction of the river, can yield camping opportunities. Soon you are in a lodgepole forest, where many sections have enough moisture to harbor denser-than-usual understory vegetation. Near some good

Panorama south from Mather Pass

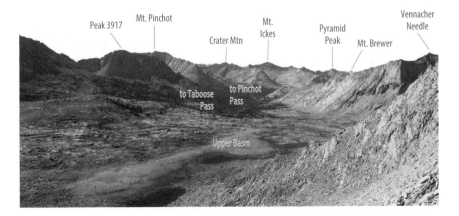

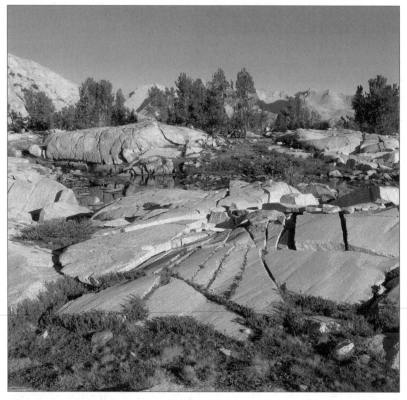

Polished granite slabs near Lake Marjorie

campsites, a rock cairn marks where an old trail, whose route you can still just follow, climbs to Taboose Pass. Farther downstream, another old and nearly vanished trail descends the South Fork of the Kings before climbing over Cartridge Pass, through Lakes Basin, and down Cartridge Creek, the route hikers used while the trails up the Golden Staircase and Mather Pass were being built. Soon you reach the main crossing of the South Fork of the Kings [10,040' – 2.3/156.7], which can be quite difficult: in early summer, you will want to wade across where the river splits around an islet downstream, and later in the season, you can hop across rocks a bit upstream. Some campsites near this crossing are closed for restoration, but options abound.

Soon after the first crossing, you ford a tributary and then begin a dry, switchbacking ascent through open lodgepole forest. One common plant on dry, south-facing slopes is Nuttall's sandwort, a straggly, matlike species with small, star-shaped white flowers and needle-shaped leaves.

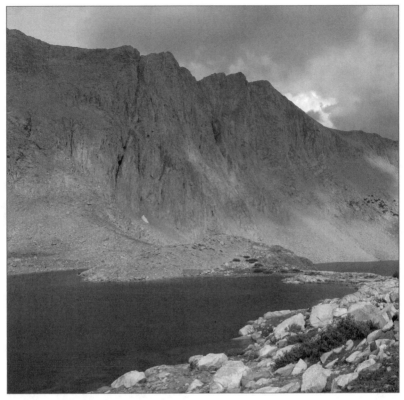

Steep walls and deep lakes north of Pinchot Pass

The steep switchbacks transition to a more gradual upward traverse, further easing as you reach a junction with the main Taboose Pass Trail [10,760' – 1.1/157.8]. Within minutes, you step across a small trickle and then ford the creek draining from Pinchot Pass. By late season, the creek banks will be decorated with the dainty brook saxifrage, with long stalks of small white flowers and round, deeply serrated leaves. Just beyond is the signed junction with the Bench Lake Trail. If you have extra energy to walk another 1.6 miles, Bench Lake, perched high above the South Fork of the Kings River, has beautiful campsites along its northeastern shore, sporting justifiably famous sunrise reflections of Arrow Peak.

A short distance south along the JMT is the Bench Lake Ranger Station, located about 0.1 mile to the north of the first lake you reach; note that this ranger station is a canvas tent that is not always staffed and is dismantled when empty, so its location can easily escape your notice. As you walk, be sure to stop and look north to Mather Pass: The

(Continued on page 166)

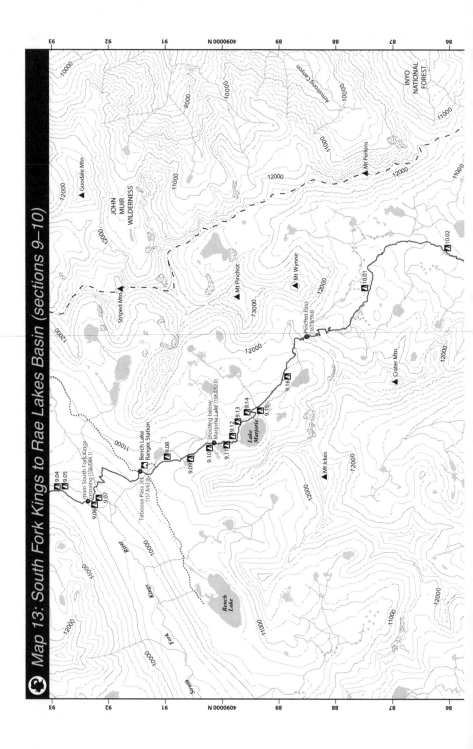

Map 13: South Fork Kings to Rae Lakes Basin (sections 9–10)

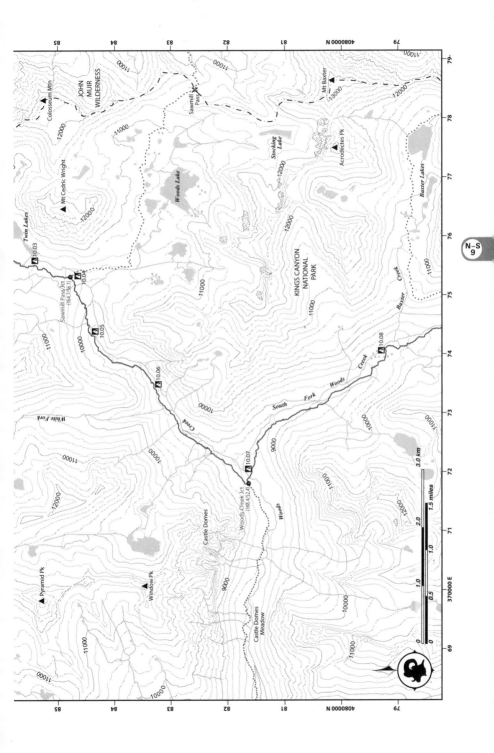

(Continued from page 163)

impressively steep peak just north of the South Fork of the Kings is Mt. Ruskin. Small campsites exist on sandy, slightly forested knobs to the side of most of the next several tarns you pass. Their outlets are all easily crossed, mostly on large blocks of rock. The final crossing is just downstream of the last tarn before Lake Marjorie [11,050' – 1.0/158.8]. Between this crossing and Lake Marjorie, you can find small tent sites tucked away in sandy patches beneath the stunted whitebark pines, including some near Lake Marjorie's outlet.

The JMT traces Lake Marjorie's eastern shore and ascends past the last krummholz. Your final miles to Pinchot Pass are very different from those ascending Mather Pass. You are in soils formed by a mixture of the dark-colored granodiorites and metasedimentary rocks, which both decompose to form a richer soil than granitic sands; water is also abundant here. Therefore, instead of switchbacking through endless blocks of big talus, you cross little creeks and meadows, which are covered by an enormous diversity of plants. A few sandy patches even provide campsites not far below the pass. On moist slopes, you will pass shrubs covered with bright yellow flowers, each of whose five petals approximate the shape of a rose petal; it is shrubby cinquefoil, a member

Panorama north from Pinchot Pass

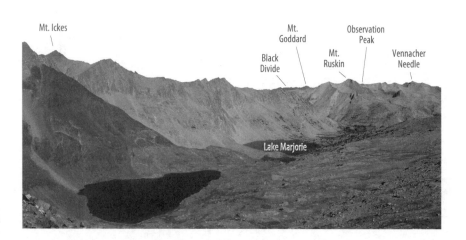

of the rose family. Wet meadows are covered with primrose monkey-flower, Sierra penstemon, little elephant's head, and tundra aster, a purple daisy, always with a single head, whose petals are incurved nearly to a point where they attach to the central disc. Small, sandy flats are covered by masses of short, red, straggly stems, the remains of early-blooming bud saxifrage. The last climb to the pass is then dominated by talus species, including many requiring wet conditions, such as the delightful Eschscholtz's buttercup, always growing in the wettest patches of sand and identified by its deeply lobed leaves. Soon you are on the summit of the pass, looking back one last time to Mather Pass and Upper Basin [12,130' – 2.2/161.0]. In contrast to steep-sided granite summits like Mt. Ruskin, the much-fractured rock here leads to peaks that are piles of loose scree. Although Mt. Wynne, directly east from the pass, is predominately composed of granodiorite, this particular pluton was one of the first to solidify and is riddled with inclusions—imbedded blobs of preexisting rock—that have been deformed and often appear as elongated ovals. The summit of Mt. Wynne, as well as Mt. Pinchot to the north and Crater Mountain to the southwest, are composed of the ancient metamorphic rocks. The small patches of white in the otherwise red rock are bits of calcite, a mineral that is rare in the Sierra.

N–S
9

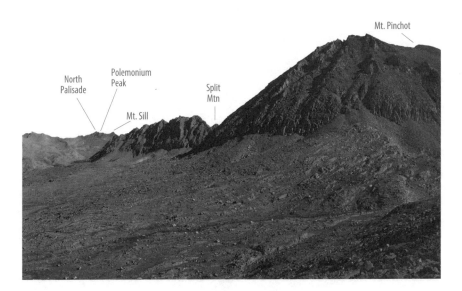

Mt. Pinchot

North Palisade

Polemonium Peak

Split Mtn

Mt. Sill

SECTION 10.

Pinchot Pass to Glen Pass: Woods Creek Fork of the Kings River (16.3 miles)

Looking south from Pinchot Pass, you take in the next magnificent alpine basin—once again meadows and little tarns surrounded by mountains. This drainage, Woods Creek, is a tributary of the South Fork of the Kings River; their confluence is in Paradise Valley, approximately 4 miles downstream of where the JMT crosses Woods Creek. Down you go on tight switchbacks, navigating through the craggy

Panorama south from Pinchot Pass

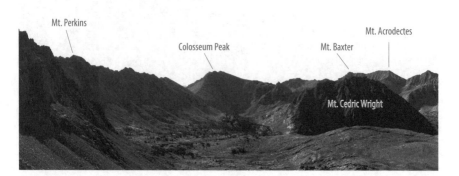

LOCATION	ELEVATION	DISTANCE FROM PREVIOUS POINT	CUMULATIVE DISTANCE	UTM COORDINATES
Pinchot Pass	12,130'	—	161.0	11S 374287E 4088510N
Sawmill Pass junction	10,350'	3.7	164.7	11S 375315E 4084786N
Woods Creek junction	8,510'	3.7	168.4	11S 371808E 4081636N
Baxter Pass junction	10,220'	4.0	172.4	11S 374516E 4077254N
Rae Lakes Ranger Station junction	10,590'	2.0	174.4	11S 375128E 4074656N
Sixty Lake Basin junction	10,560'	1.0	175.4	11S 374963E 4073712N
Glen Pass	11,970'	1.9	177.3	11S 374120E 4072254N

N–S
10

headwall below the pass, and then across flower-strewn alpine meadows, stepping across a streamlet here and there. Crater Mountain, to the west, has an amazing vista south to the King Spur if you have half a day to spare (see page 217). Once you are past the uppermost meadows, the JMT curves east to traverse above an enchanting series of ponds and lakes—if you don't have time for a break now, come back just to visit them someday. The trail once stayed in the river drainage, but now it stays high to avoid damaging the delicate meadow vegetation; you are instead traversing through short sections of talus and

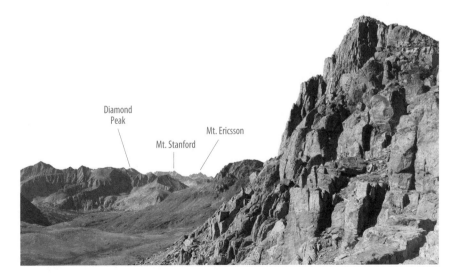

Diamond Peak

Mt. Stanford

Mt. Ericsson

rocky outcrops, interspersed by long, sandy stretches. Only once down below 11,000 feet do you skirt the edge of a small lake, where there is camping on small knobs to the east of the trail. The trail continues downward, alternatively in sections of whitebark and lodgepole forest, across slabs and sandy patches, and through dry sedge meadows. The latter are often dotted with small, yellow flowers resembling dandelions: alpineflames. Elsewhere, you may have seen the superficially similar mountain agoseris, but this species lacks the central disc seen in the alpineflames, such that the multilength ray petals converge in a single point. Some stretches of slab are splendid, with inclusions of darker rocks readily visible in the granite. A spur trail, marked only by a small cairn, leads to some secluded campsites near the outlet of Twin Lakes. You pass the signed junction to the trail northeast to Sawmill Pass [10,350' – 3.8/164.7]; a few exposed campsites lie on the bench just east of this junction, across the multistranded creek.

Descending more steeply now, the JMT drops into the sunstruck, southwest-trending canyon of Woods Creek, passing a good campsite near 9,850 feet. You next cross beneath a long talus field dotted with tall lupines, willows, fireweed, scarlet penstemon, pennyroyal, and wavyleaf paintbrush. One not-yet-mentioned species is Sierra angelica, sporting an enormous spherical head of miniature white flowers on a tall stalk. The trail now follows the creek's northern shore, often providing good views of the small stream gorge, including stretches of dashing cascades. On one bench are the first foxtail pines that you have seen; this southern Sierra species will shortly become much more common in the subalpine zone. Farther along this same bench is a collection of campsites, mostly quite small. Continuing the descent, you

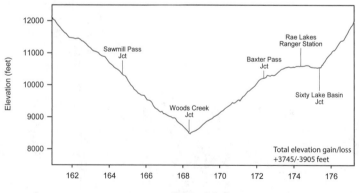

Distance (miles)

will next ford the White Fork tributary, possibly difficult in early season; consider the giant piles of boulders to either side of the creek to realize its power in flood. Around this elevation, you descend back into the realm of towering Jeffrey pines and, a bit later, western junipers as well. On the other side of the creek, you observe a well-delineated lateral moraine, the piles of material pushed to the side by a glacier that once flowed down this canyon. The trail takes you ever deeper into the canyon, crossing several more tributaries. Although these will all be wades in early summer, the crossings are flat, providing good footing on small- to medium-size rocks. Give your feet a brief break from the rocky trail and stare at the now towering walls around you, Castle Domes to the north and the King Spur to the south, and the stream cascading down smooth slabs. You now descend the final manzanita-covered slope to the trail junction with the Woods Creek Trail [8,510' – 3.6/168.4], which goes south down Woods Creek, past Paradise Valley, to Cedar Grove.

At the junction, you trend south and southeast to the overgrown north bank to cross roaring Woods Creek on an imposing, narrow, and very bouncy suspension bridge known as the Golden Gate of the Sierra. (One person at a time, please.) The bridge was completed in 1988 and is not subject to washouts like its predecessor. On the south bank, beneath Jeffrey pines, red firs, and a few lodgepole pines, is a large camping area and two food-storage boxes. South of the trail are additional campsites near a juniper-covered knob. Note that until you reach the Rae Lakes Basin, there are no more large campsites and only a few small, marginal camping opportunities. But once you reach the Rae Lakes, the campsites are mostly large and you can expect company each night. As you continue up the South Fork of Woods Creek, you pass through many vegetation communities: the first stretch is through open lodgepole forest with occasional red firs, where a cobble-covered forest floor is evidence of past flood events. Chickarees will be scampering up and down the trees, scolding you if you walk too close. This is the last lower-elevation forest you will pass through on the JMT; you will not drop below 9,500 feet until you descend east of Whitney. Higher up, the trail crosses long sections of dry, open knobs with small sedge meadows and slabs on which mountain pride penstemon, mountain big sagebrush, Nuttall's sandwort, and wavyleaf paintbrush are usually common. About 1.5 miles upstream of the Woods Creek crossing, you ford a stream draining a perched basin of lakes on the northern tip of the King Spur; the water can be deep in early summer. Another mile upstream, you pass a large, marshy meadow filled with wildflowers. By late summer, three species

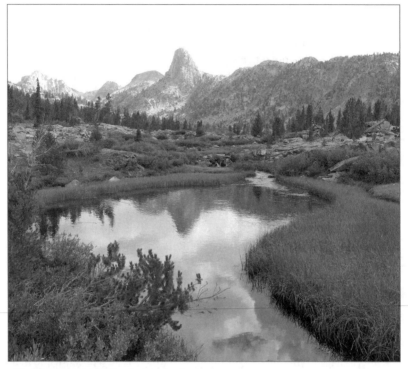

Fin Dome and the Rae Lakes Basin

of gentian will be blooming here: the stalkless, white-colored alpine gentian; Sierra gentian, with a single, narrow, tubular, purple flower on a 4-inch stalk; and the periwinkle-colored felwort, with numerous star-shaped flowers on an 8-inch stalk. By August, the alpine gentian and Sierra gentian are widespread meadow constituents throughout the Sierra, while the felwort is only common from here south. Several species of orchids, all with subtly different small, white-green flowers, are also present here. Just thereafter, you climb across a moraine and reenter the main drainage; here you find a small campsite downstream of the trail. Crossing the outlet from Sixty Lake Basin, you continue upstream and the terrain becomes ever rockier and drier. Foxtail pines slowly replace the lodgepole pines, and by the time you emerge onto granitic slabs streaked with dark-colored dikes, you are in a stark landscape of scattered foxtail pines. Their long, dangling branches often have needles only near the tip, where they encircle the stem like a bottlebrush. Where the slope lessens, you reach Dollar Lake and the junction with the Baxter Pass Trail [10,220' – 4.0/172.4].

This marks the beginning of the Rae Lakes Basin, a scenic and highly used area with a well-earned reputation for bad mosquitoes. Due to the high visitation numbers, you may only camp for two nights at each lake. There are a few campsites near Dollar Lake and more a short distance upstream at Arrowhead Lake. Both are beautiful locations with excellent sunset and sunrise reflections of Fin Dome, the prominent, steep granite dome a bit upstream. Dollar Lake is more exposed, and you camp on open, sandy patches among granite slabs; Arrowhead Lake's campsites are under lodgepole forest near a food-storage box, and the lake is ringed by a large meadow and reeds. Above Arrowhead Lake, you continue climbing through lodgepole forest.

Along your trek, you may have noted a burgundy-colored succulent, especially prominent in rocky seeps. This is western roseroot, and it also occurs sporadically in this stretch of forest. As you approach Fin Dome, the grade eases and you reach the upper basin with the three large Rae Lakes. At the lowest lake, a food-storage box and large camping area are present among scattered whitebark pines. As you traipse upcanyon, you next pass a sign marking the location of the Rae Lakes Ranger Station, a short distance east of the trail [10,590' – 2.0/174.4]. Your traverse along the east side of the lakes is lovely; you cross many little flower-filled seeps and look out across the lakes and westward to the steep peaks of the King Spur: Mt. Cotter and Mt. Clarence King. As you continue around the Middle Rae Lake, the views to the south and east become enticing as well—colorful rock, especially on the face of the Painted Lady at the head of the canyon, and the blocky outline of the Sierra Crest near Dragon Peak.

Thanks to the marshy meadows, seeps, and many lakes, birds are abundant: Yellow-rumped warblers, the all-yellow Wilson's warblers, and white-crowned sparrows are likely darting in and out of willows at the edge of meadows; Clark's nutcrackers will be congregating in whitebark pines. Near the south end of the Middle Rae Lake, a sign points you toward the lake's shore, where there is a large camping area with food-storage boxes. You cross between the Middle and Upper Rae Lakes on a narrow isthmus and, just after fording the connecting stream, you reach the junction to Sixty Lake Basin [10,880' – 1.0/175.4], a subalpine basin worth exploring if you have a few hours to spare. The lakes are exquisite, and if you walk toward the northern end of the basin, the views of the east face of Mt. Clarence King are sublime. Scattered small campsites exist west and northwest of the junction.

(Continued on page 176)

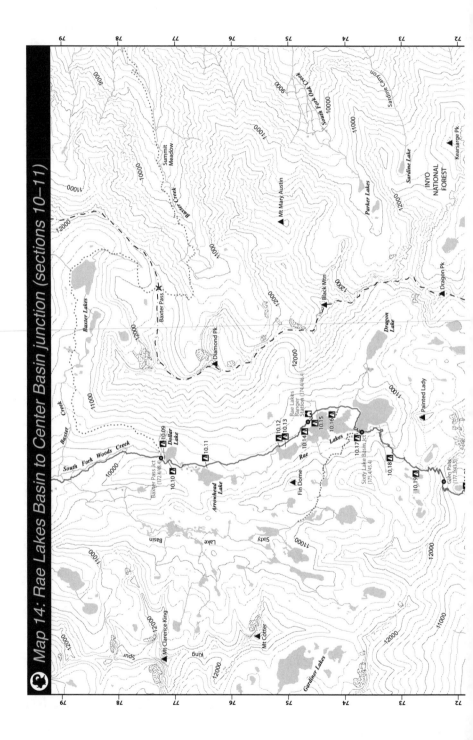

Map 14: Rae Lakes Basin to Center Basin junction (sections 10–11)

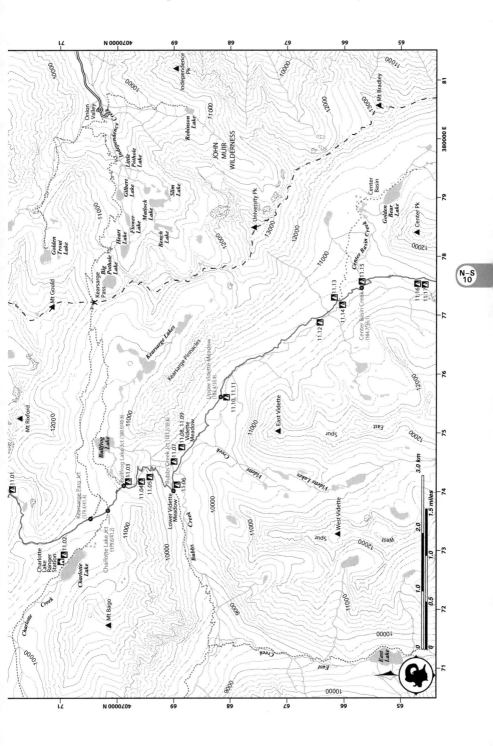

(Continued from page 173)

From this junction, you begin the switchbacking climb to Glen Pass. Keep your eyes open as you climb, as these next miles are where you are most likely to see Sierra Nevada bighorn sheep. You pass through sheep habitat several times on your journey, but the animals are both rare and difficult to spot—"boulders with legs," in the words of one researcher. However, a herd of rams is regularly spotted here atop rocky knobs or in talus; I have seen them on both my recent trips through here, and I don't often have luck seeing sheep. Your climb begins under scattered tree cover, with an understory often dominated by red mountain heather, but as you climb, you are increasingly switchbacking among slabs or next to an occasional creek. Knobs to the east of the trail provide small campsites with views down-canyon. The slope briefly flattens as you cross talus and slabs in a basin of austere mountain tarns. A few minute sandy patches may beckon to you as campsites, but, unfortunately, their exact location becomes more obvious as you continue up the trail and away from them. If you wish to detour to climb the Painted Lady, which offers an outstanding near-aerial view of the Rae Lakes, it is on this flat that you

Panorama north from Glen Pass

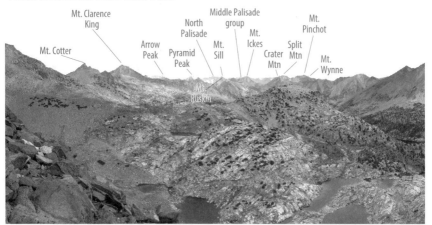

leave the trail (see page 218). The vegetation from here to the summit of Glen Pass is remarkably sparse; a few sections sport dense patches of Sierra primrose, and cracks in outcrops are again filled with dwarf ivesia, with its tufts of small yellow flowers. Three other species may also engage your eye as you continue upward: alpine mountain sorrel grows beneath shaded boulders and is identified by its rounded leaves and elongated stalks of either white flowers or red seeds; Coulter's fleabane daisy, another common member of the alpine community, has a dense head of up to 120 purple ray petals; granite (or Lemmon's) draba is a cushion plant that is ubiquitous under moist boulders. It is a type of mustard with small, four-petaled yellow flowers that cover the top of the cushion when in bloom. The higher you rise, the more often you should pause to enjoy the view northward: Great peaks dominate a barren, rocky, brown, lake-speckled world with precious little green of tree or meadow visible—and yet, having just passed through it, you know the area is rich with beautiful lakes and streams, trees, meadows, and wildflowers. Follow the last few switchbacks—which often hold snow throughout the season—until you finally land atop the narrow and windy Glen Pass [11,970' – 1.9/177.3].

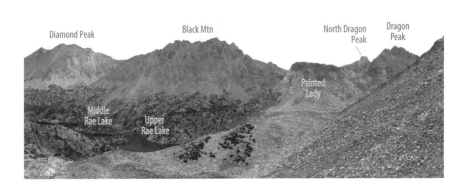

SECTION 11.

Glen Pass to Forester Pass: Bubbs Creek Fork of the Kings River (12.0 miles)

The southern side of Glen Pass drains into Bubbs Creek, another fork of the South Fork of the Kings; the two merge just upstream from Cedar Grove, approximately 18 trail miles to the west. Your view south from Glen Pass is mostly blocked by the steep-walled cirque into which you will descend. However, to the southwest, you can see the northern tip of the Great Western Divide: pyramid-shaped Mt. Brewer flanked by the unimpressive South Guard and notably steep North Guard. Switchbacks take you down a dry, loose scree slope to a couple of pothole lakes and a seasonal alpine stream. As always, the ground becomes more vegetated as the grade lessens, in this case with red mountain heather and Sierra primroses growing

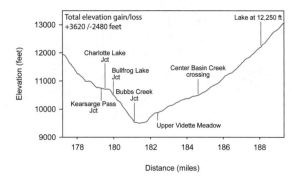

LOCATION	ELEVATION	DISTANCE FROM PREVIOUS POINT	CUMULATIVE DISTANCE	UTM COORDINATES
Glen Pass	11,970'	—	177.3	11S 374120E 4072254N
Kearsarge Pass junction	10,770'	2.1	179.4	11S 373545E 4070469N
Charlotte Lake junction	10,740'	0.2	179.6	11S 373685E 4070166N
Bullfrog Lake junction	10,520'	0.4	180.0	11S 374109E 4069887N
Bubbs Creek junction (Lower Vidette Meadow)	9,550'	1.2	181.2	11S 374026E 4069006N
Upper Vidette Meadow food box	9,910'	1.2	182.4	11S 375616E 4068174N
Center Basin Creek	10,530'	2.3	184.7	11S 377469E 4065704N
Lake at 12,250 feet	12,240'	3.4	188.1	11S 377813E 4062539N
Forester Pass	13,110'	1.2	189.3	11S 377379E 4061665N

N–S
11

among boulders. A few small tent sites are nestled among the white-bark pines on the southwest side of the first lake. You descend more switchbacks to a second lake, this one a depression completely surrounded by talus and lacking an outlet; it is quite possibly the only lake along the JMT that lacks any acceptable campsite. As you pass it, look southeast at the steep-fronted pile of talus, as this is another rock glacier.

The trail soon curves west, enters sparse lodgepole forest, and, before long, trends south. You are now perched high above Charlotte Lake and have extensive views to the west: Charlotte Dome is the steep, polished dome downstream, and Mt. Bago is the large mountain at the southern end of Charlotte Lake. The summit of Mt. Bago provides the views to the Kings-Kern and Great Western divides that were lacking from Glen Pass. If you wish to summit Mt. Bago, take a detour at the Charlotte Lake junction a short ways downslope (see page 218). You continue your traverse across a dry slope dotted with foxtail pines and reach a junction to Kearsarge Pass [10,770' – 2.1/179.4]. If you must exit to the Onion Valley Trailhead and the town of Independence to resupply, take this branch. Just a short distance downstream, you enter an enormous sandy flat, in the middle of which is the Charlotte Lake junction, also known as Sandy Junction [10,740' – 0.2/179.6]. There is ample camping, a food-storage box, and a ranger station at the northeastern end of

Charlotte Lake, 0.9 mile along the spur trail. Alternatively, heading east from this junction also takes you to Kearsarge Pass.

Leaving the sandy flat behind, you ascend briefly through white-bark and lodgepole pines, cross an exposed knob with foxtail pines, descend a short, steep slope with rocky footing, and reach yet another junction that leads to Kearsarge Pass—this one via Bullfrog Lake and the Kearsarge Lakes Basin [10,520' – 0.5/180.0]. There is a small tent site near the junction, but camping is prohibited at Bullfrog Lake, and stock are prohibited on this trail. The JMT continues dropping south into the Bubbs Creek canyon. While the descent is mostly through steep, dry lodgepole forest, there are small, flat campsites near two creek cross-ings. At each of the stream crossings, you pass the expected collection of species: Coulter's fleabane daisy, great red paintbrush, Kelley's tiger lily, arrowleaf ragwort, California corn lily, and swamp onion. Half-way down, where the trail briefly exits the forest, you are on a slope covered with bush chinquapin and are likely looking across the canyon to the steep face of East Vidette, an arête that formed where the glaciers descending Vidette Creek and Bubbs Creek merged. There are large, shady campsites at the Lower Vidette Meadow Trail junction [9,550' – 1.1/181.2], where the Bubbs Creek Trail continues downstream to Roads End at Cedar Grove, while the JMT resumes its upward march.

The trail meanders along the flat, dry forest floor, crossing the out-let from Bullfrog Lake, a ford that can be a wade in early summer. The forest is nearly barren—for long stretches, the upright pods of rockcress are all you see, and underfoot are large cobbles deposited here by past floods. The trail now leads past Vidette Meadow, where there are large campsites and a food-storage box beneath lodgepole pines. There is also an excellent view of the northeast face of East Vidette. The trail briefly emerges onto a steeper, open slope before leveling out near Upper Vidette Meadow. Here, there are additional food-storage boxes and good campsites, both along the main creek and near the several tribu-taries you cross [9,910' – 1.3/182.4]. Now the grade becomes gradual to moderate, and the forest cover thins as you ascend beside the won-derful cascades and pools of upper Bubbs Creek. For long stretches, the landscape is covered with downed tree limbs—evidence of past avalanches. Fireweed and low-growing willows are pioneer plants in this landscape. Due to this disturbance, your views are open; be sure to look up at the steep walls of East Vidette and southward to Center Peak, yet another arête. After this long stretch with limited camping options, you finally reenter open lodgepole forest. Shortly thereafter, you pass a small cairn and note a conspicuous line of rocks indicating

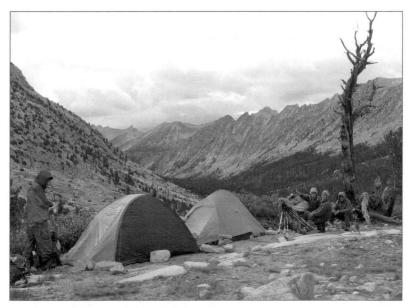

Camping high above Bubbs Creek

the start of a trail, the only remaining marker for the still easy-to-follow trail to simply lovely Center Basin. Although now unmaintained, this was initially going to be the route of the JMT; a route across the Kings-Kern Divide (via Forester Pass) had not yet been found and the trail was to be routed through Center Basin, across Junction Pass (east of Junction Peak), down to the *east* side of Shepherd Pass, and finally back over Shepherd Pass to near the Tyndall Creek crossing. Just beyond are large campsites and a food-storage box. A short distance later, you ford Center Basin Creek [10,530' – 2.2/184.7], which can be high in early summer, and pass the last forested campsites for many miles.

You quickly leave the lodgepole forest behind. By now, you are familiar with the subalpine landscape: Scattered whitebark pines dot the scenery; where there are small streams, the ground is marshy and the vegetation includes mountaineer shooting stars, dwarf bilberry, little elephant's heads, Lemmon's paintbrush, and primrose monkeyflower, with lupines and felwort adding new colors later in the summer; where you cross dry slabs or drier sedge meadows, wide-leaved Parish's yampah, alpineflames, pussypaws, and Sierra penstemon dominate. Above a series of small creeks, there are campsites on sandy, whitebark pine-covered knobs, all with spectacular views

(Continued on page 184)

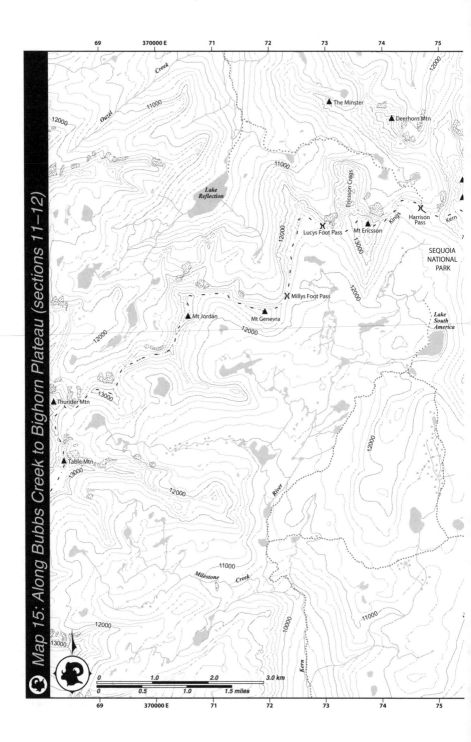

Map 15: Along Bubbs Creek to Bighorn Plateau (sections 11–12)

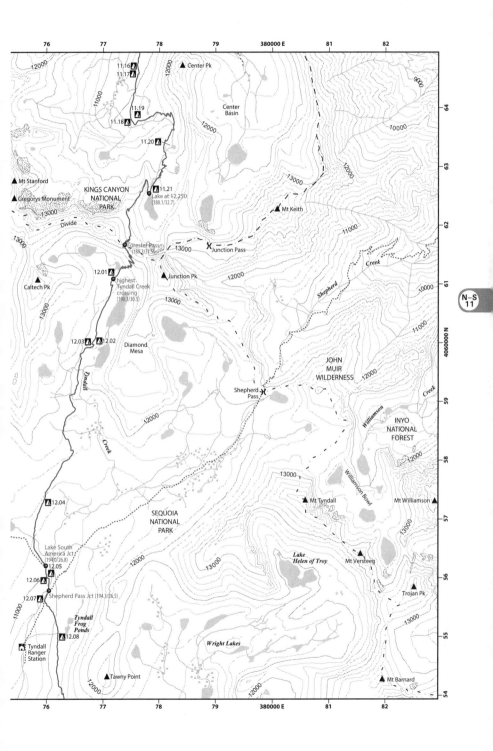

(Continued from page 181)

up and down Bubbs Creek: To the southwest is the vertical face of Mt. Stanford, and to the south is the steep Kings-Kern Divide. You pass more meadows, creeks, and, increasingly, piles of talus. This is the land of the alpine chipmunks and pikas. These small, round members of the rabbit family with adorable Mickey Mouse ears emit a two-noted "cheep-cheep" when disturbed. Most impressively, this species does not hibernate in winter, but lives beneath talus piles, eating hay that it has prepared in summer. At 11,230 feet, you pass the last clump of whitebark pines and another small campsite. There is another even more exposed campsite at the edge of the next meadow, with even more magnificent views, of course.

It is difficult to imagine that you have left the last tree behind, yet you still have nearly 2,000 feet to climb to Forester Pass. As you continue your climb into the alpine zone, you will see occasional sandy tent spots among meadows and slabs. As always, please be sure to camp in previously used locations to limit your impact on resources in this fragile area. Moving rocks exposes the roots of the small alpine plants, causing them to desiccate and likely die. The JMT strikes east across an alpine meadow and just to the side of the shallow, gravelly creek that is the headwaters of Bubbs Creek. Then it climbs a short stretch of moist switchbacks, where the Eschscholtz's buttercup and

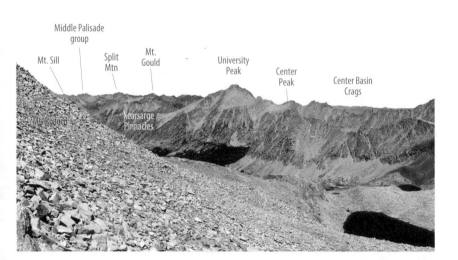

alpine mountain sorrel are both common, and emerges on one last meadow and a slab-strewn bench. This landscape is home to water pipits, spotted sandpipers, and gray-crowned rosy finches. Water pipits and spotted sandpipers are both especially common in Center Basin with its expansive wet, hummocky, alpine meadows. If you are lucky, you may see a golden eagle soaring high above the mountains. You are also now back in the realm of light-colored granite, having left the darker-colored granodiorites and red-hued metamorphic rocks behind when you descended from Glen Pass. Only one strip of "odd-colored" rock now decorates the landscape; look east to a pile of dark-colored talus—this so-called mafic plutonic rock is part of the same material that comprised the Painted Lady; it solidified underground, just like granite, but has far more dark-colored minerals and little to no quartz and feldspar.

The remainder of the climb is now through talus, and here you will, for the first time on the JMT, see abundant specimens of the Sierra's two classic alpine species: skypilot and alpine gold. Skypilot has unmistakable 3-inch-diameter, deep purple heads of tubular flowers, and alpine gold is a large yellow daisy with remarkably sticky stems and leaves. But probably most remarkable about these two is their size; in marked contrast to the fell-field species you have seen over the 12,000-foot passes, both of these plants are 4–8 inches tall. And to think they both only grow at these high elevations. Climbing up near the crest of an old

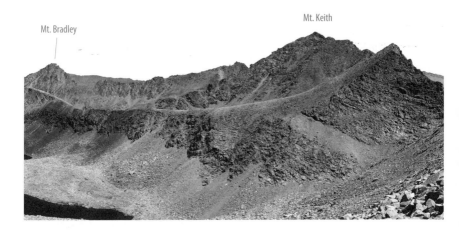

Panorama north from Forester Pass; photographed by Brad Marston

moraine, you reach the outlet of Lake 12,250 (or 12,090 on older maps) [12,240' – 3.5/188.1]. Barren and stark, there are some small tent and bivvy sites in the talus to the east of the outlet, with the potential for a beautiful sunset view of Junction Peak reflecting in the lake.

Just below the outlet, where the water mostly flows beneath the talus field, you cross the creek one last time. You now ascend a narrow ridge and enjoy your last views toward Mt. Stanford. As you continue, look back at Center Peak: the summit looked so tall and imposing as you began your climb from Vidette Meadow, yet soon you will be higher than the summit. You now commence the final southward traverse and ensuing switchbacks, where snow may linger very late. On the north side of this pass there are often no visible plants—most species cannot grow during the brief, snow-free weeks, and you will probably only see the dark-colored heads of Heller's sedge emerging next to boulders.

Forester Pass is atop the Kings-Kern Divide, the border between the Kings River drainage that you have been traversing since Muir Pass, and the Kern River drainage to the south. While the Kings River has many east–west trending forks, resulting in one high pass after another, the Kern River runs north–south and therefore the next stretch of the JMT has fewer long descents and ascents. Instead, you find yourself climbing in and out of many small canyons and then, of course, up the slopes of Mt. Whitney. This high pass is also the border between Kings Canyon and Sequoia National Parks. And a word of warning: Enjoy the views from the north side of the pass, as the south side is quite a wind tunnel [13,110' – 1.2/189.3]!

SECTION 12.

Forester Pass to Trail Crest: Kern River (23.2 miles)

The view from the top of Forester Pass is breathtaking and vast: To the southwest are the dark, jagged summits of the Kaweahs; to their east, the long, straight fault scarp through which flows the Kern River; and straight ahead, the magnificent rolling tundra landscape through which you will next walk. As you stare down the steep southern side of Forester Pass, you will not be surprised that trail engineers had initially planned to route the JMT elsewhere. However, by 1931, just a year after its discovery, this pass had been scouted and built, streamlining the route south to Whitney. In winter, however, skiers still use creative route-finding to successfully cross this divide. Now you descend numerous exposed switchbacks, some of which are cut into the rock, and others of which are built atop stone walls. Growing on this near-vertical cliff face are dwarf ivesia, as always, sticking out from

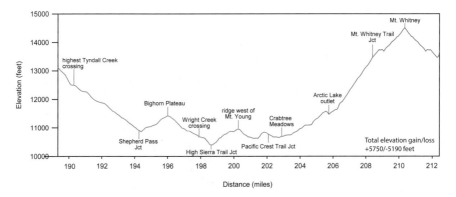

LOCATION	ELEVATION	DISTANCE FROM PREVIOUS POINT	CUMULATIVE DISTANCE	UTM COORDINATES
Forester Pass	13,110'	—	189.3	11S 377379E 4061665N
highest Tyndall Creek crossing	12,500'	1.0	190.3	11S 377175E 4061080N
Lake South America junction	11,040'	3.7	194.0	11S 375992E 4056208N
Shepherd Pass junction	10,910 '	0.3	194.3	11S 376045E 4055781N
Bighorn Plateau	11,430'	1.7	196.0	11S 376685E 4053326N
Wright Creek crossing	10,680'	1.9	197.9	11S 377085E 4050965N
High Sierra Trail junction	10,410'	0.8	198.7	11S 377431E 4050541N
ridge west of Mt. Young	10,960'	1.6	200.3	11S 377126E 4048918N
PCT junction west of Crabtree Meadows	10,770'	1.8	202.1	11S 378213E 4046605N
Crabtree Meadows and Crabtree Ranger Station	10,700'	0.8	202.9	11S 379241E 4047243N
Arctic Lake outlet creek crossing (Guitar Lake)	11,470 '	2.9	205.8	11S 382513E 4048029N
Mt. Whitney Trail junction	13,460'	2.6	208.4	11S 384376E 4046713N
Mt. Whitney summit	14,505'	2.0	210.4	11S 384473E 4048700N
Trail Crest	13,670'	2.1	212.5	11S 384493E 4046577N

Panorama south from Forester Pass; photographed by Brad Marston

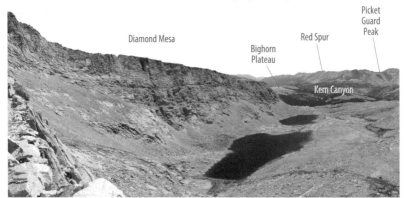

cracks. A bit lower is abundant magenta-colored, large-flowered, four-petaled rockfringe, growing from the base of boulders and outcrops. Toward the bottom, you pass a monument to Donald Downs, a trail crew member who died during the trail's construction. After igniting dynamite for trail work, he and others hid behind large boulders to the side—a standard practice. Unfortunately, rocks above and around them shook loose, pinning Donald's arm and injuring three others. The large boulder was successfully removed, but his arm was shattered. A doctor was called to the scene and his arm amputated, but unfortunately, an infection set in and took the 18-year-old's life before he was able to be evacuated. It is a good reminder of the effort and dedication required to produce what we now take for granted. (The plaque is located at approximately 12,500 feet, UTM 11S 377418E 4061491N; it is easy to miss while traveling south.) Where the grade eases are small, exposed sandy patches that fit a tent. Just thereafter, you cross the nascent Tyndall Creek for the first time [12,500' – 1.0/190.3].

You now begin a delightful walk down the broad, gentle valley. The scale of the headwaters of the Kern is difficult to get used to after walking through the more-intricate terrain to the north; it feels more like a desert landscape, where you can walk several miles and feel as if you are in nearly the same location. To the east, the steep faces of Junction Peak and Diamond Mesa are incongruous; they stand out all the more noticeably in comparison to the gentle sandy grade underfoot. The summits of these peaks were never glaciated, and the steep, smooth chutes on their western faces are all the result of avalanche activity; only the lower reaches of the peaks bear signs of past

N–S
12

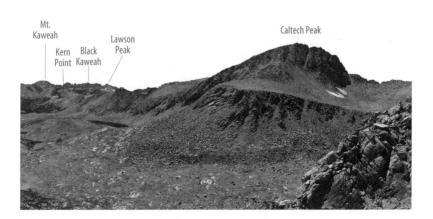

Mt.
Kaweah

Kern Black   Lawson
Point Kaweah   Peak   Caltech Peak

glaciation. For many miles, you wander through this sandy landscape, dotted by boulders and alpine tarns of all sizes, and with abundant fell-field species covering the ground. Three different species of buckwheat share this area: the yellow-flowered frosted wild buckwheat that has been common on all dry substrates from the montane to the alpine; the white- to pink-flowered Sierra cushion wild buckwheat, whose leaves bear such dense hairs that they appear nearly white; and Coville's sulphur flower, a yellow-flowered species with spade-shaped leaves and long flower stalks lying horizontally on the ground. Growing so close to the ground allows these plants to avoid the persistent wind chill and to maintain leaf temperatures warmer than the surrounding air. And look up as well, for in the distance, you get your first view of Mt. Whitney, the tall, flat-topped peak with large avalanche chutes on its northern face.

The trail passes through one small stand of mixed lodgepole and foxtail pines, where there is a campsite, and shortly reaches a signed junction for the Lake South America Trail, taking you to a beautiful basin and the true headwaters of the Kern River [11,040' – 3.7/194.0]. Both the views from the lake and the surrounding landscape make it one of my favorite places in the Sierra; it is well worth a half-day detour. Admiring the beautiful cluster of foxtail pines to the west, you soon reach the Tyndall Creek crossing and camping area (with food-storage box); please camp in the locations specified by the ranger and note that in the Kern drainage, campfires are now prohibited above 10,400 feet, which includes just about the entire trace of the JMT. The Tyndall Creek crossing may be short, but the fast-flowing, freezing-cold water and rocky bottom make it formidable in early summer. In a few more steps, you pass the Shepherd Pass Trail, the Sequoia National Park side of which was rebuilt in 2006 to skirt marshy areas in the valley [10,910' – 0.3/194.3]. Next, you pass a junction for the trail that heads down Tyndall Creek. The often-unstaffed Tyndall Creek Ranger Station is 0.6 mile down this trail—much farther than is shown on many maps. There are campsites at the junction. After passing the three trail junctions in rapid succession, you can avoid navigating for a number of miles: Head south (left) and uphill, following zigzags toward the Tyndall Frog Ponds where there are large campsites, a food-storage box, warmish swimming, and beautiful views of Diamond Mesa.

You continue climbing, skirting around the western side of Tawny Point, first through dry lodgepole forest, then onto drier, more exposed slopes that are dominated by foxtail pines, and eventually onto a barren flat of sand, the monotony broken only by tufts of sedges and mounds

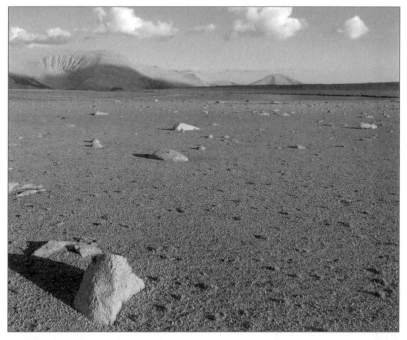

Bighorn Plateau

of matted Brewer's lupine. The views, however, keep opening up; not only can you see the country you have just traversed to the north, but also ever more of the Great Western Divide. From south to north are Milestone Mountain, a narrow pinnacle; Midway Mountain, a not-too-inspiring peak; Table Mountain, with vertical sides and a flat top; and Thunder Mountain, a steep and imposing pyramid. Where the trail crests is a nearly round tarn [11,430' – 1.7/196.0]. This is Bighorn Plateau, named for sheep once seen to the east. Ironically, the plateau itself is lousy sheep habitat, as the sheep stick to cliffy areas where they can outmaneuver predators. Sandy, flat, unvegetated patches make for possible campsites, and their views speak for themselves. Take special note of Mt. Whitney, which now has a prominent position on the skyline to the southeast. Plan ahead to spend some time here, as the location is magical: Early in the morning, you'll likely hear packs of coyotes; a few hours later, you can watch the ravens sitting in the foxtail pine snags; American kestrels and other birds of prey will soar above you; and marmots will sun themselves on nearby boulders. In case the view

(Continued on page 194)

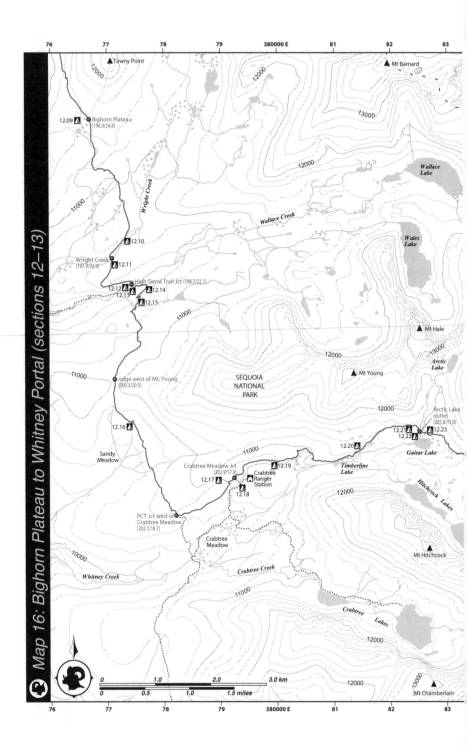

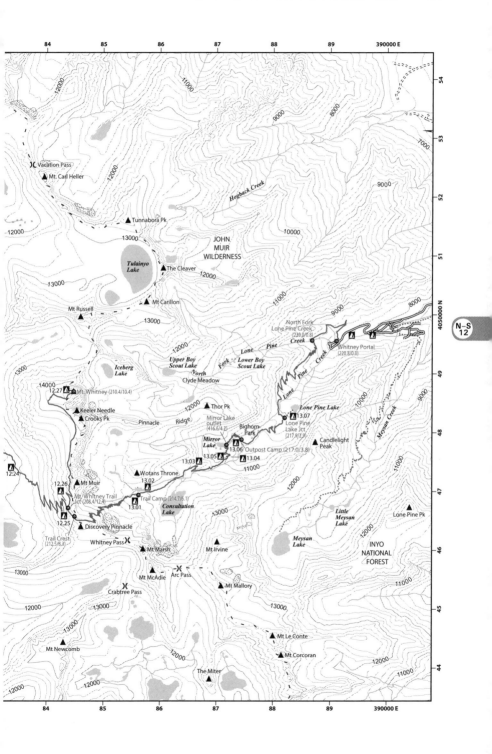

(Continued from page 191)

isn't quite good enough, climb up Tawny Point for the full panorama (see page 219), or wander westward to one of the shorter knobs overlooking the Kern drainage.

After Bighorn Plateau, the JMT descends into the Wright Creek drainage. A hardscrabble sandy slope marks the remnants of an old moraine. Elsewhere, the trail skirts the top of long meadows with small streams, tributaries of Wright Creek filled with Bigelow's sneezeweed, a wild sunflower with big, bright, yellow flowers and dark "noses." In late summer, the stragglier-looking orange sneezeweed takes center stage. A few campsites present themselves as you drop into lodgepole forest, and you'll encounter a much better one just after you ford the main Wright Creek. This crossing may be difficult in early summer, as the water can be deep [10,680' – 1.9/197.9]. Another short climb follows, and you cross a forested flat, reach the lip of the Wallace Creek drainage, enjoy yet another vista to the Kaweahs, and descend on a dry, sandy slope to the High Sierra Trail junction [10,410' – 0.7/198.7]. The High Sierra Trail begins at the Giant Forest in western Sequoia National Park and now follows the same path as yourself, all the way to the summit of Mt. Whitney. Just beyond the junction is the Wallace Creek crossing, which can also prove difficult in early summer, for although the rocks underfoot are small, it is a long crossing. On the south bank are popular campsites and a food-storage box.

Yet again, the JMT heads uphill, this time skirting around the giant west shoulder of Mt. Young, en route to Crabtree Meadow. A few switchbacks up, you cross a creek, beside which is one small tent site. The climb began in lodgepole forest, but as soon as the slope gets steeper, foxtail pines become dominant. As you ascend, note that the granite you pass is pinkish due to potassium feldspar, one of the minerals in granite. Here it is easily visible, as the granite has a higher percentage of potassium feldspar and the individual rectangular crystals are large. Elsewhere, note greenish surfaces on fractured boulders; this is the mineral epidote, which commonly fills small cracks in granite. Throughout the climb, enjoy the artistic trees interspersed with large boulders and a filtered view across to the Kaweah Peaks. Where the slope eases, the foxtail pines again give way to lodgepole pines and you reach the apex of the shoulder [10,960' – 1.6/200.3]. The ensuing traverse and slight descent lead to the edge of Sandy Meadow, which the JMT skirts along its upper edge. There is one campsite toward the eastern side of the meadow, but note that there may be no late-season

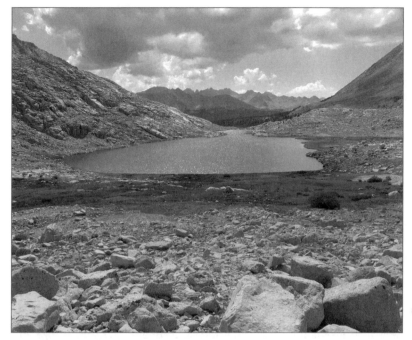

N–S
12

Guitar Lake with the Kaweah peaks behind

water here. The forest floor is bare, save scattered individuals of a few species, including Sierra penstemon and Nuttall's sandwort. In contrast, the banks of each little trickle you cross are densely covered, and here you find primrose monkeyflower, carpet clover, Parish's yampah, ranger's buttons, and much more. Hopefully you are not yet too tired of this lumpy topography, as there is one more ascent ahead, up to a ridge radiating southwest from Mt. Young, followed by a descent to a trail junction, where the PCT and JMT part company for good. The PCT continues south from here to the Mexican border (and the route to Cottonwood Pass and the Cottonwood Lakes), but you turn eastward for your last ascent of the trip: up nearly 4,000 feet to the summit of Mt. Whitney [10,770' – 1.8/202.1].

The JMT heads east, along a dry bench with scattered foxtail pines and, at times, a view to the summit of Mt. Whitney. After you enter denser forest cover, pass one campsite, and ascend a zigzag, you reach the Crabtree junction [10,700' – 0.8/202.9]. Turning right takes you to the Crabtree Ranger Station, a food-storage box, and a selection of campsites. Mt. Whitney is straight ahead. Also at this junction is a large box containing human waste bags that all hikers bound for Whitney

Portal are required to use once east of Timberline Lake, a short distance ahead. If you didn't receive one when you began your hike, please take and use one to preserve the water quality and pristine landscape for all future hikers (see the section on water purification and camp hygiene on page 34 for additional information).

You continue upward following a river terrace on the north shore of Whitney Creek, passing first through open lodgepole forest (with several campsites) and then increasingly walking across dry, open slopes. The latter are covered with shaggy hawkweed, ocean spray, wavyleaf paintbrush, pennyroyal, granite gilia, and, for the first time since Thousand Island Lake, the periwinkle-colored western blue flax. A stemless white thistle is dinnerplate thistle, the stalked deep red thistle is rose thistle, and the yellow-rayed daisy with shiny, non-hairy serrate leaves is western dwarf mountain ragwort. A set of switchbacks up slabs takes you to Timberline Lake, where camping is prohibited, but photographing Mt. Whitney mirrored in its still waters is encouraged. You'll pass one small campsite, nestled among willows above Timberline Lake. As your climb continues, to your left is a dry, sandy slope, and to your right is various meadow and creek-side vegetation. Beneath rocks is pink alumroot and occasionally Sierra primrose and rockfringe, while red mountain heather covers large expanses of sandy substrate, doing a remarkable job of holding the loose material in place. By August, the strips of wet meadow will be dotted with white Sierra gentians and purple alpine gentians. When the trail levels out into a wet-sandy flat, you are nearly at Guitar Lake. Here, you can leave the trail to find campsites above the "guitar's neck," or you can continue up the trail to Arctic Lake's outlet [11,470' – 2.9/205.8] for additional camping. All sites have beautiful views of the evening alpenglow on the west, the now-hulking face of Mt. Whitney, and good morning light in the direction of the Kaweahs. Be sure to fill your water bottles here, as in some years, it is the last water until Trail Camp, nearly 10 miles away on the other side of Mt. Whitney.

After skirting the meadow at the inlet of Guitar Lake and passing two small tarns, your final 3,000-foot (!) climb begins. You first climb up sandy, bouldery slopes, crisscrossed by seeps, many of which are filled with both Bigelow's sneezeweed and orange sneezeweed. Just below 12,000 feet, you reach a bench, dotted with small seasonal ponds and edged with slabs. There are fantastic views from this bench down to the Hitchcock Lakes, across to Mt. Hitchcock, and, of course, expansive views westward. And on the slabs, a short distance west of the trail, you will find the last large campsites before Mt. Whitney. Now you

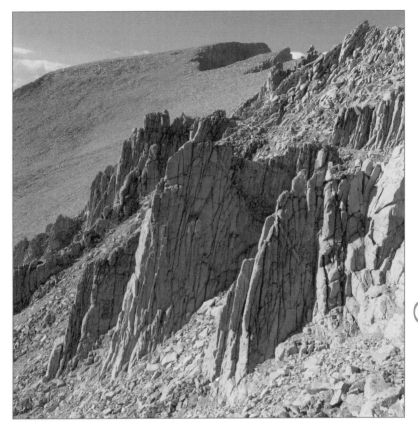

The final traverse to the summit of Mt. Whitney

find yourself on endless switchbacks in increasingly barren talus. You'll notice that the granite here is very light-colored—there are few dark crystals—and that the rock contains large, rectangular feldspar crystals. If you're lucky, you'll see ones embedded with dark, rectangular outlines of minuscule dark minerals, showing where other minerals began to grow but were engulfed by a single, ever-expanding feldspar crystal; this is called a zoned crystal. Upward you climb, now in the realm of the rosy finches and ravens. Skypilot and alpine gold are abundant here, joined by a few other hardy species, Sierra primrose, rockfringe, Western dwarf mountain ragwort, granite draba, alpine mountain sorrel, dwarf ivesia, Coulter's fleabane daisy, and another daisy with three-lobed leaves, cutleaf fleabane daisy. Sometimes its central yellow disc is rimmed by purple ray petals, and other times these are absent. As you continue higher, evermore species disappear from the mix, until only skypilot, alpine gold, and granite draba are common. As you finally approach the Mt. Whitney Trail junction, you note a few austere and windy, but view-rich and dramatic bivvy and tent sites, where boulders have been used to build small walls and the sandy area in between can hold a small tent. Suddenly, you reach the trail junction [13,460' – 2.7/208.4] and intersect the vast quantities of human traffic headed for Mt. Whitney's summit: On most summer days, 150 people receive either a day-use or overnight permit to ascend the peak from Whitney Portal.

Most JMT hikers leave their overnight packs (or at least most of its contents) at this location, carrying only water, food, a jacket, and, of course, a camera, to the summit. (But note, the marmots are hungry too, so lock your food-storage canister.) Although you are well-acclimated, take these last miles slowly. Don't push yourself so hard that you need constant breaks, but instead find a pace that allows you to keep oxygen intake in balance with exertion. You climb first up a talus slope. For a long stretch, the trail then winds past notchlike windows with views down to the east and among pinnacles, the tallest of which is Class 3–4 Mt. Muir, another 14,000-foot peak. It is a beautiful peak and an exhilarating climb, but didn't John Muir deserve more than a subsidiary peak of that named for his nemesis, Josiah Whitney? (Whitney was the state geologist who contested Muir's analysis that there was widespread evidence of past glaciation in the Sierra Nevada.) The trail then emerges on one final giant, barren, talus slope, and passes two even taller, but much less steep pinnacles, Crooks Peak (previously known as Day Needle) and Keeler Needle, which is considered insufficiently distinct from Mt. Whitney to be called a peak. The trail now becomes rockier and the footing uneven as you curve around to the west and then complete the final switchbacks east to the summit, arriving at the metal-roofed summit building and the enormous summit register [14,505' – 1.9/210.4]. From there, you will undoubtedly head east to the true summit, marked by a metal plaque. Unless a storm threatens, give yourself a good long break on top—you have just completed the JMT! Walk around the entire summit plateau, as there is a unique view in each direction. Especially stunning is the vista down the east face of the mountain, to Trail Camp and Consultation Lake, and beyond to the town of Lone Pine, 10,000 feet below. The end of your trip lies some 6,000 feet below, so retrace your steps to the junction and turn east, leaving the official JMT, and continuing for 0.15 additional mile to the highest pass on this journey, Trail Crest [13,670' – 2.1/212.5].

Sunrise from Mt. Whitney

Many people decide to end their trek by watching sunrise from the summit of Mt. Whitney. Having had the same goal on many occasions, I can attest to the amazing experience of watching the sky slowly turn from black, to gray, to pale morning colors, and then the sudden explosion of color and warmth as the first rays of sun hit you. If this is how you wish to complete your journey, here are a few ways to reach the summit in time and a few points to ponder:

• **Contemplate** whether you're prepared to spend the night at 14,505 feet; it will be cold and even though you are now well acclimated, this is a very high camp. If you wish to camp on the summit, you should carry 3–4 liters of water per person, for you need enough both to cook dinner and breakfast, as well as to complete the 9.2 miles of walking between Guitar Lake and Trail Camp. Expect nighttime temperatures to drop below 0, especially if there is any wind. Do not depend on the summit cabin for shelter.

N–S
12

• **If you camp at Guitar Lake,** you will need to complete the most strenuous 4.7 miles of the JMT in the dark—and miss out on seeing the views from this section. Even though you are well acclimated, give yourself 3–5 hours to complete this stretch, for you will move slower in the dark and would hate to miss the sunrise by 15 minutes!

• **Another option** is to spend the night at one of the bivvy sites high on Mt. Whitney (Camps 12.25 and 12.26). You still need to carry up your water, but you will be camping 1,000 feet lower and can complete the final miles without your pack. You will also get to see the entire trail in the daylight.

• **As a final alternative,** summit in the afternoon, enjoy the late-afternoon light, and then descend to Trail Camp for the night. In the morning ascend Wotans Throne (see page 220) to watch the sunrise on the east face of Mt. Whitney.

I have tried each of these options on Mt. Whitney or other Sierra peaks, and they are each exquisite and rewarding but with slightly different advantages and drawbacks.

Panorama southeast from Mt. Whitney

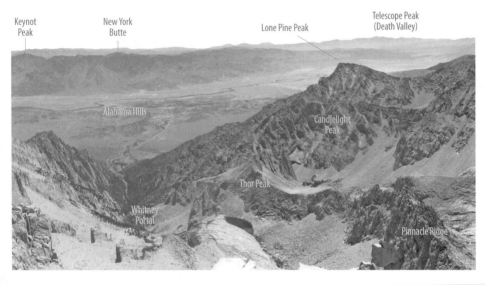

Panorama southwest from Mt. Whitney

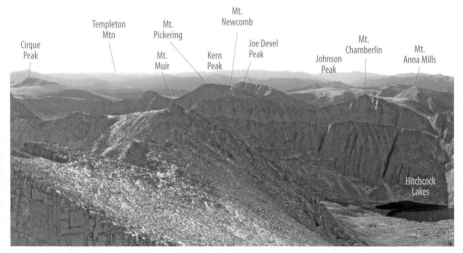

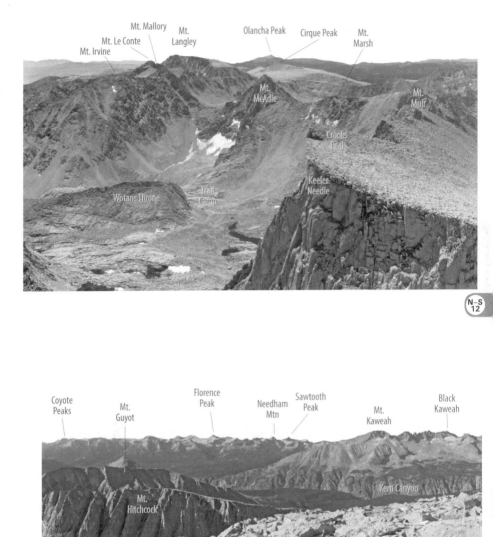

N–S
12

Panorama northwest from Mt. Whitney

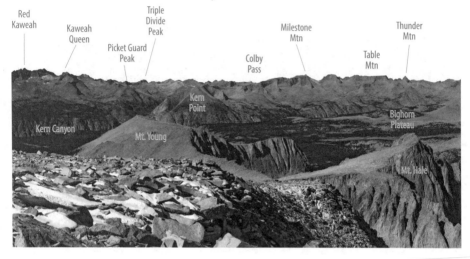

Panorama northeast from Mt. Whitney

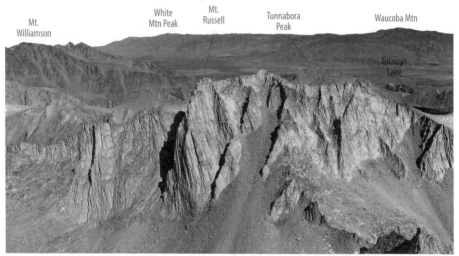

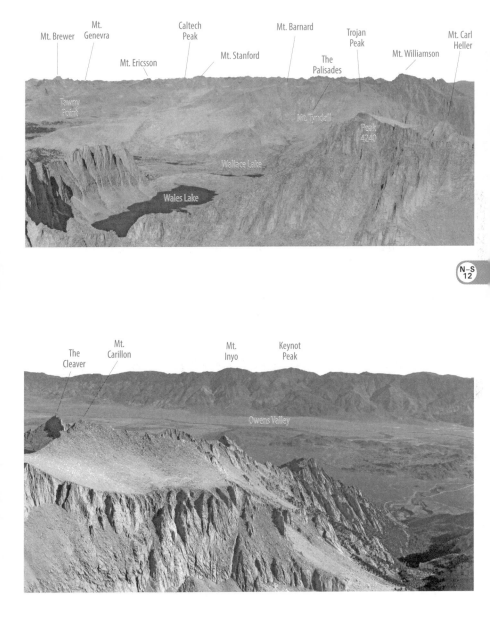

Mt. Brewer Mt. Genevra Mt. Ericsson Caltech Peak Mt. Stanford Mt. Barnard The Palisades Trojan Peak Mt. Williamson Mt. Carl Heller

Tawny Point Mt. Tyndall Peak 4240

Wallace Lake

Wales Lake

N–S 12

The Cleaver Mt. Carillon Mt. Inyo Keynot Peak

Owens Valley

SECTION 13.

Trail Crest to Whitney Portal: Owens River (8.3 miles)

At Trail Crest, you leave Sequoia National Park and enter John Muir Wilderness. You are now in the Lone Pine Creek drainage, which flows into the Owens River, dead-ending in Owens Lake. You are at the top of a steep, talus slope, this one laced with just under 100 tight switchbacks; after an initial traverse, back and forth you go down the northeast-facing slope. About two-thirds of the way down is a section where the trail has been blasted into a cliff. Here, water seeps through cracks, and this section is notorious for being ice-covered long into summer. Fortunately, there is a cable you can cling to if necessary. The

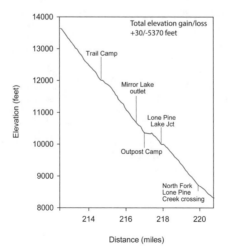

LOCATION	ELEVATION	DISTANCE FROM PREVIOUS POINT	CUMULATIVE DISTANCE	UTM COORDINATES
Trail Crest	13,670'	—	212.5	11S 384493E 4046577N
Trail Camp	12,040'	2.2	214.7	11S 385616E 4046956N
Mirror Lake outlet	10,670'	1.9	216.6	11S 387181E 4047813N
Outpost Camp	10,370'	0.4	217.0	11S 387445E 4047888N
Lone Pine Lake junction	10,010'	0.9	217.9	11S 388197E 4048255N
North Fork Lone Pine Creek crossing	8,720'	2.1	220.0	11S 388672E 4049562N
Whitney Portal	8,330'	0.8	220.8	11S 389136E 4049566N

long descent ends at Trail Camp [12,040' – 2.2/214.7]. Here, tent sites have been created in every flat spot available among the pervasive slabs and boulders, and there are many places to camp on both sides of the trail. One thing, however, is missing from this alpine perch: a good view of the east face of Mt. Whitney; the large moraine rising straight above camp in combination with Pinnacle Ridge to the south block the view of Mt. Whitney. This can be remedied by an early-morning ascent of Wotans Throne, the peak immediately south of Trail Camp that is a straightforward climb from its northern or northwestern side (see page 220). I advocate a predawn start, so you can watch the sunrise on Mt. Whitney's east face. After nearly completing your journey, this may not sound appealing, but after 50 other campers and many day hikers start tromping around and through camp in the wee hours, why not get up and enjoy the morning light?

You now have just 6 miles to go! You descend a rocky granite trail, crossing Lone Pine Creek, and passing now-familiar flowers such as rockfringe, alpine prickly currant, ocean spray, and granite gilia. The thornless currant is the wax (or squaw) currant, and is likewise abundant. Along rock faces is rosy-petaled cliffbush, under rocks is Sierra primrose, and where it's wetter are the larger mountain and primrose monkeyflowers. You pass one small campsite just before you reach small, wet Trailside Meadow (camping prohibited), through which Lone Pine Creek flows. This area is filled with brightly colored mountaineer shooting stars. The first trees appear around 11,000 feet, at which point there are simultaneously stunted foxtail and lodgepole pines. Some switchbacks later, past a few small campsites, the trail finally flattens out at Mirror Lake, where camping is prohibited [10,670' – 1.9/216.6]. You cross its outlet and proceed downward across a dry, south-facing slope covered with bush chinquapin, wavyleaf paintbrush, pennyroyal, shaggy hawkweed, mountain pride penstemon, and scarlet penstemon. At the bottom of the slope lies Outpost Camp [10,370' – 0.4/217.0], a second large camping area beneath tall foxtail pines. The trail curves southeast along the upper edge of the adjacent marshy area, Bighorn Park. Leaving this area, you climb slightly before descending switchbacks to a large, sandy flat covered with Sierra mousetail and home to some quite tame pikas. Here, you'll spot the sign marking the end of the Mt. Whitney Zone. Around the corner is the lateral to oddly under-filled Lone Pine Lake, at which there are camping possibilities [10,010' – 0.9/217.9].

From here, you have only 2.5 miles to go. But as you race downward thinking about home, or maybe a hamburger, or perhaps wishing to turn around and hike back northbound, take time to look at the steep, white granite walls on either side of the canyon and the view down Lone Pine Creek. You descend through open lodgepole forest to a log crossing over Lone Pine Creek. Your exposed descent continues down yet another long set of switchbacks. The lower you get, the less familiar the vegetation is; for the first time on your journey, you encounter the mid-elevation, dry, eastside chaparral community: curl-leaf mountain mahogany, with its white, twisted "seed tails" and in-rolled leaves; singleleaf pinyon pines; and fern bush, a tall shrub with fernlike leaves and white flowers. Below, you cross the main branch of the North Fork of Lone Pine Creek [8,720' – 2.0/220.0], which can be difficult in early summer, as well as a small tributary. You then walk your final steps to Whitney Portal, where you can weigh your now nearly empty backpack [8,330' – 0.8/220.8]. Congratulations, you've made it!

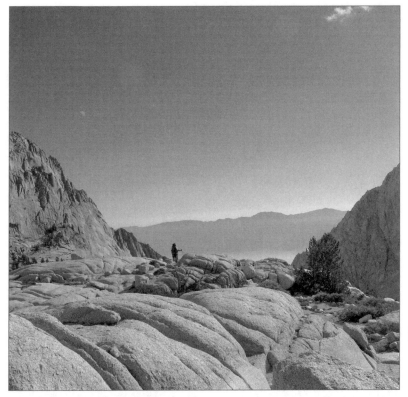

Crossing slabs on the descent to Whitney Portal

N–S
13

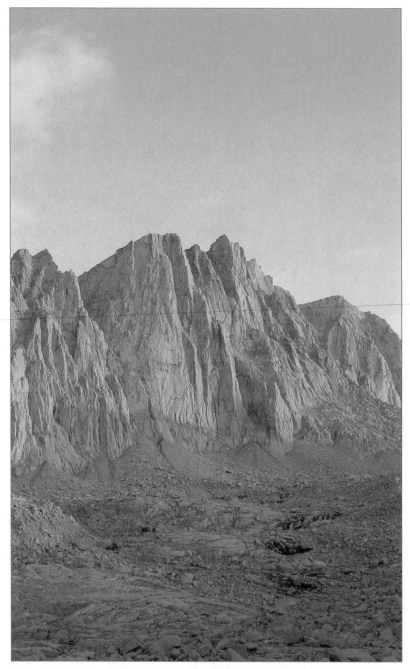

The skyline from Trail Camp with Mt. Whitney on the far right

SIDE TRIPS TO PEAKS, VISTA POINTS, AND LAKE BASINS

More than 100 named summits lie within 2 miles of the John Muir Trail, and many have nontechnical ascent routes. Described here are just 15 of them, chosen for their views, the straightforward route-finding to their summits, and, in many cases, for the absence of large amounts of loose talus. Few of the peaks described in this section are the tallest or most prominent in an area, but don't feel short-changed. The best views of a basin are usually from the slightly shorter peaks that lie in the middle of basins, rather than the tallest peaks that grace the crest.

If this is the first time you are hiking off-trail to ascend peaks, do not be intimidated, just cautious. As indicated in the time estimates, hiking off-trail is much slower than trail travel; I estimate a little more than 1 hour per mile, throwing in a bit extra for breaks. For the stretches of these routes that are on talus, take your time and don't trust a rock that is precariously balanced on others. One advantage of the Sierra is that you can usually see your entire route due to the lack of tree cover at high elevations, but you should still carry a map and compass to navigate safely.

If you plan to bag many summits while hiking the JMT, I recommend that you bring along a more exhaustive reference, such as R. J. Secor's *High Sierra: Peaks, Passes, and Trails* or Steve Roper's *The Climber's Guide to the High Sierra*. However, if your schedule will allow just an occasional free afternoon to climb a peak, this selection is more than sufficient. If you depart from the JMT at a junction listed in the cumulative mileage table on pages 62–65, just the distances from Happy Isles and Whitney Portal are given (100.0/120.8). If your departure point is between junctions, both the mileage and the UTM coordinates are given.

One word of warning: Bears are also active during the day, and you are legally required to protect your food at all times, so remove your food-storage canister from your pack, lock it, and stash it in the shade any time you embark on an excursion.

Peaks and Vista Points

Section 1

Half Dome

Elevation: 8,836'
Elevation Gain/Loss: ±1,800'
Round-Trip Distance: 4 miles
Round-Trip Time: 4 hours

Climbing Half Dome has become nearly as much of a John Muir Trail requirement as summiting Mt. Whitney. A permit is now required to hike Half Dome, and you must request one together with your wilderness permit; receiving one is no longer guaranteed for backpackers. Once at the Half Dome junction (5.9/214.9), remove, lock, and stash your food-storage canister in an unseen location and then separately hide the rest of your pack, before proceeding up the Half Dome Trail. The first mile and a bit are through forest, and you then emerge on the granite slabs of Half Dome's "shoulder." The trail that ascends the first section of slabs is remarkable—the switchbacks are so well-constructed that you focus only on the steep steps, not the underlying slabs. A short descent brings you to Half Dome's famous cables. Take a breather, and proceed upward. Comfortingly, as with all domes, the slope lessens the higher you get and the way down is much easier than you expect it to be. Enjoy the view down into Yosemite Valley and to the Yosemite high country. For a map of the trail, see Map 1 on pages 70–71.

Clouds Rest

Elevation: 9,926'
Elevation Gain/Loss: ±1,920'
Round-Trip Distance: 7.9 miles
Round-Trip Time: 5 hours

The north face of Clouds Rest is a nearly 5,000-foot granite slab rising above Tenaya Canyon. While this peak is much less popular than Half Dome, its extra 1,000 feet of elevation provide hikers with an even more stunning view of the Yosemite high country, as well as an excellent view of Half Dome. From the Forsyth Trail junction (8.6/212.2), turn north and then northeast, climbing steadily up a forested slope alongside a fork of Sunrise Creek. Continue up through forested terrain to a T-junction (2.4 miles from the Forsyth junction), where you turn left (west) and climb gently up a dry, sandy ridge. At a second junction just before the summit, stay north (right) and climb onto the quite steep summit ridge. Follow it west to the summit. You can also ascend to the summit from the Clouds Rest junction, but that route is slightly longer. For a map of the trail, see Map 1 on pages 70–71.

Columbia Finger shoulder

Elevation: 10,220'
Elevation Gain/Loss: ±280'
Round-Trip Distance: 0.75 mile
Round-Trip Time: 1 hour

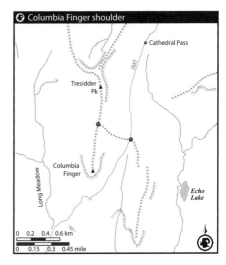

The Cathedral Range includes many strikingly steep pinnacles and ridges of granite because the constituent Cathedral Peak granodiorite has few fractures and is very resistant to weathering. This also means that all of the summits you pass along the JMT are quite technical; Columbia Finger is one of the easiest, but even its summit requires some exposed scrambling at the top. Therefore, instead of ascending one of the peaks, I have included a viewpoint that surrounds you with summits: the ridge that connects Columbia Finger and Tresidder Peak. Between Long Meadow and Cathedral Pass, the trail surmounts a ridge (15.7/205.1; 11S 287307E 4188741N). From this high point head west cross-country up through forest and broken slabs to the ridge. From the summit you will have a splendid view of Tenaya Peak, Matthes Crest—an impressively steep, mile-long fin of rock—and the Echo Peaks.

Section 2

Lembert Dome

Elevation: 9,450'
Elevation Gain/Loss: ±800'
Round-Trip Distance: 2.3 miles (add 2.2 miles if starting at campground)
Round-Trip Time: 2–3 hours

Lembert Dome is a popular walk for all hikers visiting Tuolumne Meadows. The hike begins at a parking lot along the Tioga Road, 0.4 mile east of the wilderness permit office (23.6/197.2; 11S 294373E 4194605N).

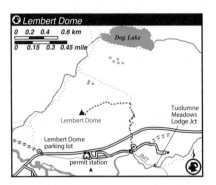

The trail climbs north, crossing CA 120, and continues up steep switchbacks through forest to a junction after 0.6 mile. Head left to climb up the ridge to Lembert Dome. After 0.4 mile, the trail reaches the saddle between the two summits and vanishes. From here, follow slabs south to the summit. Lembert Dome is an excellent vantage point for the Tuolumne Meadows area, with views of Mt. Dana and Mt. Gibbs to the east, Lyell Canyon to the south, and the Cathedral Range and Tuolumne Meadows to the west. (On your return trip, you can either retrace your steps, or at the trail junction east of the summit turn left and continue north. The trail loops north around Lembert Dome, ending at the Lembert Dome parking area, a nice loop if you started your excursion at the campground.)

Donohue Peak or Donohue Pass vista

Elevation: 12,023'
Elevation Gain/Loss: ±1,200'
Round-Trip Distance: 3.3 miles
Round-Trip Time: 3–4 hours

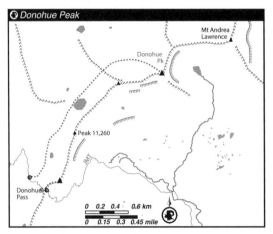

The top of Donohue Peak is a bit of a talus slog, but with an excellent view down Lyell Canyon, south to the Ritter Range, and into the San Joaquin drainage. Starting about 0.25 mile west of (and 150 feet below) Donohue Pass (35.8/185.0; 11S 301782E 4181720N), head cross-country north across granite outcrops, traversing gently across Peak 11,260 to reach a lake just to the north. (You can also begin at Donohue Pass, but this will add about 200 feet of elevation gain and loss to your journey.) From the lake head northeast up and across the face of Donohue Peak, ascending the northwest face once you are well around the ridge; this slope is gentler than the western ridge of the peak. Although the top section of this route is mostly talus, the talus is quite stable. The first ascent of the peak was made on horseback from the northwest. If you have time for just a quick detour, the knob (11S 302171E 4181578N) that rises just 0.1 mile north of the pass has a much more expansive view than you have at the pass itself. From the pass, climb up any of the granite slabs or sandy passageways to the north, climbing just 80 feet of elevation to reach the top.

Section 4

Red Cones

Elevation: 9,032' (southern cone), 9,000' (northern cone)
Elevation Gain/Loss: ±170' (southern cone), ±370' (northern cone)
Round-Trip Distance: 0.5 mile (for each)
Round-Trip Time: Less than 1 hour

The Red Cones are a pair of cinder cones on either side of the Crater Creek crossing, near the northern of two trails to Mammoth Pass. Both sport excellent views of the Ritter Range and the John Muir Trail as far north as Donohue Pass. While the northern, and shorter, cone, is less vegetated near the summit, I prefer the view from the southern, taller cone. To reach the northern cone, leave the JMT at the creek crossing (62.2/158.8) and ascend anywhere along the cone's southwestern flank. The easiest ascent of the southern cone is made if you continue 0.4 mile farther south along the JMT

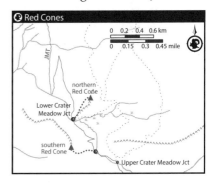

(62.6/158.4; 11S 318644E 4161815N), stopping just before a small creek crossing. From here head due west, first across a quite even landscape and then climbing steeply to reach the summit. The best vista points are slightly west of the summit. For both peaks, whenever possible find a slightly less direct and less steep route to minimize the frustration of "two steps climbed up, one step slid back down."

Section 6

Volcanic Knob

Elevation: 11,140'
Elevation Gain/Loss: ±1,400'
Round-Trip Distance: 3.5 miles
Round-Trip Time: 4–5 hours

Volcanic Knob requires a bit more of a detour and more complex route-finding than most peaks listed, but it is well worth the walk past

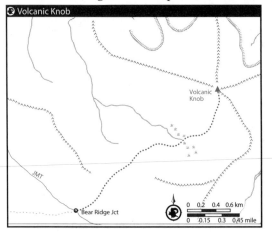

two hidden meadows to a phenomenal vista point. This peak should not be attempted unless you are carrying a compass or GPS, as the peak is not visible from where you leave the JMT. To reach Volcanic Knob, leave the JMT at the Bear Ridge Trail junction (92.6/128.2). Head cross-country along a use trail up a small gully, trending northwest toward the southern edges of the two meadows. In the first, you will find a snow survey cabin and automated weather station. Heading east–northeast, pass over the small ridge to the second meadow and begin your climb of Volcanic Knob. The walking is easiest if you trend a bit south, to the right side of the peak, staying in the trees. Taking this route, you will encounter no talus. From the summit, you have a view northward of the Silver Divide and Silver Pass, to the west of Lake Thomas Edison, and to the south to Recess Peak, Seven Gables, and Selden Pass.

Section 7

Mount Spencer

Elevation: 12,431'
Elevation Gain/Loss: ±1,500'
Round-Trip Distance: 2.5 miles
Round-Trip Time: 3–4 hours

Mt. Spencer is one of the lowest peaks in Evolution Basin, but its central position provides excellent views in all directions, especially of the west faces of Mt. Darwin and Mt. Mendel. Leave the JMT at

Sapphire Lake's outlet (125.1/95.7; 11S 349525E 4112936N), cross the outlet stream, and head cross-country up the westerly spur extending from Mt. Spencer. This spur leads to the southern end of Mt. Spencer's summit ridge (at approximately 12,200 feet). The route takes you up polished granite slabs, giving you a first-hand feel for glacial action; avoid wet

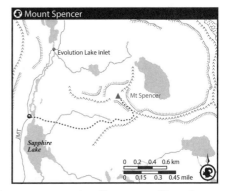

rock and take care not to slip. You then pass two small tarns and head right (south) of steep bluffs, soon reaching the skyline. From here, head north along the west side of the ridge on slabs, blocks, and sandy patches among the rocky outcrops. Nowhere is the route exposed or dangerous; if you are uneasy about the terrain ahead, look to the other side of the ridge and in places walk right along the ridge itself.

Section 8

Black Giant

Elevation: 13,330'
Elevation Gain/Loss: ±1,700'
Round-Trip Distance: 3.0 miles
Round-Trip Time: 4–5 hours

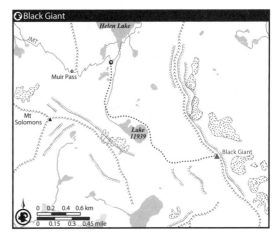

The Black Giant lives up to its name: a giant mound of dark rock stands taller than any peaks to the south or west for a long distance, providing a stunning view—to the south is a seemingly endless sea of peaks and valleys all the way to Mt. Whitney and the Kaweahs. Remarkably, a Class 1 route leads up the Black Giant, indicating easy walking with minimal talus. Head up the stream (trickle!) between not-yet-visible Lake 11,939 and Helen Lake; this is about 0.6 mile east of Muir Pass (129.7/91.1; 11S 352200E 4108563N). The landscape is full of small lumps; always aim for the lowest of them to avoid unnecessary elevation loss as you approach the lake. Skirt Lake 11,939 along its northern and eastern shores, heading for the shallow pass to its south. Just before you reach the pass, begin ascending the far southern section of the Black Giant's western slope; the easiest walking is where a slight ridge is visible. Trending due east brings you to the summit. Afternoon lighting is best, and be sure to leave yourself ample time to just sit and gaze at the scenery.

Section 9

Split Mountain or Red Lake Pass

> **Elevation:** 14,042'
> **Elevation Gain/Loss:** ±2,500'
> **Round-Trip Distance:** 4.5 miles
> **Round-Trip Time:** 6–7 hours

Besides Mt. Whitney, Split Mountain is the easiest 14,000-foot peak you will pass on the John Muir Trail. Once you have reached the flattish terrain below Mather Pass, continue another 0.3 mile (5–10 minutes) until you can head due east cross-country to skirt around the southern shore of Lake 11,595 (152.3/68.5; 11S 370608E 4098606N). Ascending and descending small lumps of granite that separate sandy expanses, you will curve around to the eastern shore, bypassing a small spur, and then turn sharply east as soon as the terrain allows. Now head up well-vegetated slopes straight toward the low point on the Sierra Crest you could see from below. (If climbing to the summit of Split Mountain is too much of a detour for your itinerary, consider climbing to Red Lake Pass. At just 12,630 feet, this is significantly less

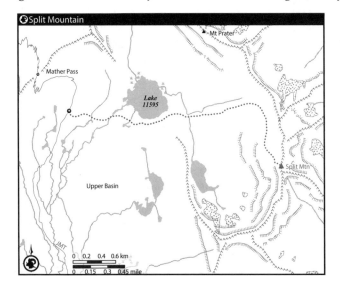

elevation and already sports a spectacular view. Here I am referring to the actual pass between Prater and Split Mountains, not the route used to descend to Red Lake.)

As you climb toward the crest you will note that in places there are bands with vegetation (tiny!) and elsewhere pure rock; when given the choice, always head for the vegetation, for the rocks in the vegetated area are always more stable and usually smaller. Continue bending around to the south and climb up the long talus slope heading to the summit of Split Mountain. In stretches there are use trails, while elsewhere you are on talus. On the lower stretches the best use "trails" are toward the eastern side of the slope, while for the final 400 feet, the best options are farther west, with no obvious cross-over choice except a band of talus. Note that you cannot see the summit until you are quite close, but it never gets any harder; just keep up the slow and steady pace and search for stripes of the easiest rock to navigate. From the top enjoy a view eastward to the Inyo and White Mountains, and the Owens Valley and expansive views of the Sierra in all other directions. Especially impressive is staring 10,000 feet down the eastern escarpment!

Section 10

Crater Mountain

Elevation: 12,874'
Elevation Gain/Loss: ±1,400'
Round-Trip Distance: 1.8 miles
Round-Trip Time: 3–4 hours

The summit of Crater Mountain has open vistas to Mt. Clarence King in the south and the White Fork of Woods Creek to the west. While loose, metamorphic rock lies near the summit of the peak, the going is much easier than on nearby summits, including Mt. Pinchot, Mt. Perkins, and Mt. Ickes. From approximately 11,500 feet on the south side of Pinchot Pass (162.0/58.8; 11S 374664E 4087689N),

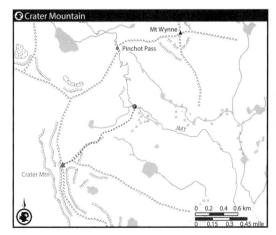

head cross-country toward and then up the northeastern spur of Crater Mountain; the rock is much more stable than in the bowl to the north. The ridge leads to a false summit, with the high point just 50 feet farther west along a narrow ridge. The traverse is neither difficult nor exposed, but stop here if you feel uncomfortable continuing. And from the second summit do not head south along the narrow craggy spur; it really is composed of dangerously loose rock. If you stop at the first summit, note that, although the view toward Mt. Clarence King, the steep pyramid just south of Woods Creek, is obstructed from this location, you have quite a good view just 200 feet back down the ridge.

Painted Lady

Elevation: 12,119'
Round-Trip Elevation Gain/Loss: ±750'
Round-Trip Distance: 1.2 miles
Round-Trip Time: 2 hours

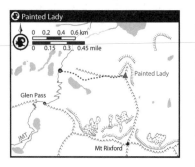

If you are willing to put up with lots of talus, you will be rewarded with a fantastic view of the Rae Lakes from the summit of the Painted Lady. Just 500 feet down the north side of Glen Pass is a flat, talus-laden basin dotted with small tarns (176.6/44.2; 11S 374371E 4072740N). From this point, head east cross-country to the Painted Lady. The initial traverse across a seemingly flat landscape to the base of the peak is the slowest, as you climb over endless pieces of colorful talus, some metamorphic and the rest altered granitic rocks. Climb along the west spur toward the steeper talus that ascends the final 500 feet to the summit. You will encounter more stable rock if you stick a little south of the west rib. From the summit, enjoy the view east to Dragon Peak and north to the Rae Lakes.

Section 11

Mount Bago

Elevation: 11,870'
Elevation Gain/Loss: ±1,050' from JMT
Round-Trip Distance: 3.0 miles from Charlotte Lake junction
Round-Trip Time: 4 hours from JMT

Mt. Bago stands alone, with no tall peaks for several miles in most directions. This location guarantees excellent views, especially to Charlotte Dome (to the west) and the Great Western and Kings–Kern Divides (to the south). Starting along the spur trail to Charlotte Lake (179.6/41.2), head west cross-country across the broad meadows and flats and then up the forested and sandy slopes toward the lower, eastern summit of Mt. Bago. A short stretch of loose gravel lies just below the ridgeline. Follow the nearly flat ridge south to the higher

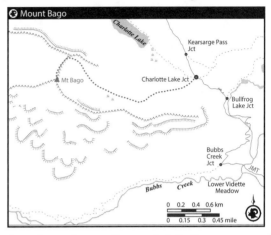

summit. The pyramid-shaped peak to the southwest is Mt. Brewer, flanked on either side by South Guard and North Guard. Due south is the very rugged Kings–Kern Divide.

Section 12

Tawny Point

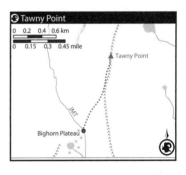

Elevation: 12,332'
Elevation Gain/Loss: ±900'
Round-Trip Distance: 1.5 miles
Round-Trip Time: 2 hours

Tawny Point is an easy hike from Bighorn Plateau, with exquisite views of the entire Kern Basin. If you climb just one peak while hiking the John Muir Trail, this is my recommendation. From the Tyndall Creek crossing south to the western Crabtree junction, you are walking along a shelf to the east of the Kern River; however, nowhere along the trail gives you a feel for the length and expanse of the river drainage. The view from Tawny Point superbly rectifies this problem; from the summit you can stare into the remarkably straight Kern drainage, west to the rugged peaks of the Kaweahs and the Great Western Divide, north to the upper Kern along the Kings–Kern Divide, and southeast to the Mt. Whitney area. As for the route, from Bighorn Plateau (196.0/24.8), head slightly northeast cross-country and then north up the southern slope of Tawny Point. There are no route-finding obstacles, with much of the route vegetated and just short stretches of easy talus a short distance below the summit.

Section 13

Wotans Throne

Elevation: 12,726'
Elevation Gain: ±700'
Round-Trip Distance: 1 mile
Round-Trip Time: 2 hours

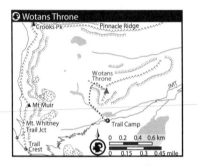

Wotans Throne has a superb view of the east face of Mt. Whitney, especially at sunrise. If you have just hiked the trail north to south and are camped at Trail Camp for your final night, this is a worthwhile detour before heading down to Whitney Portal. From Trail Camp (214.7/6.1), head north cross-country just to the right of the inlet creek above Trail Lake, staying left of the steep slabs. Where the slope of the drainage lessens, head west (left) onto the crest of the rock glacier—despite the deceptive appearance from below, this will lead you to easy walking terrain. Continue north until you are at the northwest corner of the peak. Ascend slabs and talus at either the northwest corner or the northern face to reach the summit. Avoid the temptation to start ascending too early, or you will encounter much steeper terrain.

Lake Basins

The following lake basins, all reached by trails or use trails, are excellent extras. Because they are a short distance off the JMT, they receive very little traffic, providing a different sense of solitude—and of course a different view.

Rose Lake   Trail heads south from the Rose Lake junction. (section 6; 99.3/121.5; 2 miles round-trip)

Bench Lake   Trail heads west from a junction just south of the Taboose Pass junction. (section 9; 157.9/62.9; 11S 371958E 4091327N; 3.3 miles round-trip)

Center Basin   An unmaintained, but easy to follow, trail heads north at a cairn just north of the Center Basin food-storage box. At the first tarn you reach, continue north and east around the marshy meadow to climb to Golden Bear Lake and the upper basin. (section 11; 184.3/36.5; 11S 377257E 4066066N; 4 miles round-trip)

Lake South America   From the Lake South America junction, head 0.7 mile west. At a second junction turn north, cross a wet lake basin, climb up a slope, and skirt west and north to reach the lake. (section 12; 194.0/26.8; 6.5 miles round-trip)

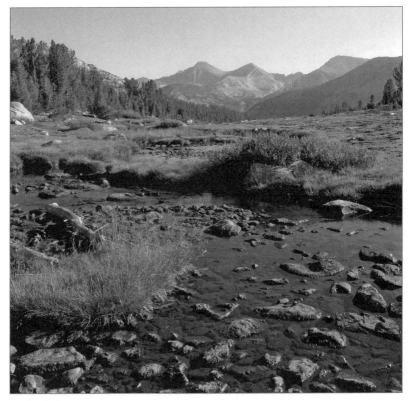

Rose Lake

APPENDIX A

JMT LATERAL TRAILS AND NEARBY TOWNS

This appendix includes information on the lateral trails diverging from the John Muir Trail to trailheads and the main towns near these trailheads. You may need to use JMT lateral trails for a variety of reasons—to resupply on food or to bail out if a member of your party is sick or injured, or if you are section hiking the trail. In general, exiting the JMT, including resupplying food, becomes more difficult the farther south you are. There are many relatively easy options in the northern third of the trail; a few long, but well-graded and well-maintained options in the middle third of the trail (including Mono Pass, Piute Pass, and Bishop Pass to the east and Lake Edison, Bear Creek, and Florence Lake to the west); and only one fairly easy eastside pass south of Bishop Pass: Kearsarge Pass. Toward the south, two of the trails heading out to the west side, Woods Creek and Bubbs Creek, are good trails with virtually no elevation gain (heading west), but keep in mind that the western trailheads are farther from population centers and finding a ride back to your car (or public transit) may prove difficult or expensive.

This section is not just for preplanning. You should at least carry a copy of the lateral trail table with you, for you cannot predict when you will have to exit the JMT due to an injury or sickness, and many JMT maps do not show lateral trails all the way to the trailheads.

JMT Lateral Trails

This section describes trails that lead from the JMT to trailheads, organized from north to south along the JMT. It does not include use trails or other cross-country routes (for example, Italy Pass) or most of the routes where the nearest trailhead is more than 20 miles distant (for example, Goddard Canyon/Hell for Sure Pass or the High Sierra Trail). If you know in advance that your route will include considerable time on some of the lateral trails, you may choose to consult other Wilderness Press books, including *Sierra North*, *Sierra South*, and *Sequoia & Kings Canyon National Parks* for additional details.

First is a table that includes basic information about each of the trails, including towns accessed, its length, elevation gain/loss (starting from the JMT), and distance along the JMT. Also included is the agency in whose jurisdiction the trailhead is and the trailhead for which you need to obtain a permit if you are beginning a section hike at this trailhead.

See page 12 for details on how to obtain permits from each park or forest.

Additional information, including trailhead amenities and a brief trail description with locations of campsites, is written for each trail, organized north to south from where it leaves the JMT; if you are hiking from your car to the JMT, the description needs to be reversed. The description also tells you how to reach the trailhead by car. Each write-up indicates topographic maps covering the route, where *USGS* indicates a U.S. Geological Survey 7.5-minute topo and *TH* indicates a Tom Harrison map.

> Abbreviations:
> NP = National Park
> NF = National Forest
> SEKI = Sequoia and Kings Canyon National Parks.

Glacier Point via the Panorama Trail (section 1)

Access to: Glacier Point, just south of Yosemite Valley (11S 273226E 4178502N)

Trailhead Amenities: Toilets, water, snacks, and bus service to Yosemite Valley

Getting to the Trailhead: From the western end of Yosemite Valley, head south on CA 41 for 9.2 miles, passing through the Wawona Tunnel and eventually reaching a left-hand junction. Turn left onto Glacier Point Road (going straight leads to Wawona), and follow it for 15.3 miles to its end at the Glacier Point parking lot.

(Continued on page 227)

TRAIL	TRAIL LENGTH	ELEVATION GAIN/LOSS	TRAILHEAD ELEVATION	JMT JUNCTION	N-S	S-N	PERMITS	TOWNS ACCESSED	PAGE
Glacier Point*	5.5	+1,710', -530'	7,200'	Panorama Trail junction	2.8	218.0	Yosemite NP: Glacier Point to Little Yosemite Valley	Yosemite Valley, Glacier Point	223
Cathedral Lakes	0.1	+0', -20'	8,560'	trail to Cathedral Lakes Trailhead	20.6	200.2	Yosemite NP: Cathedral Lakes	Tuolumne Meadows	227
Lyell Canyon**	0.0	+5', -0'	8,645'	Tuolumne Meadows permit station	23.1	197.7	Yosemite NP: Lyell Canyon	Tuolumne Meadows	227
Rush Creek	9.0	+500', -2,950'	7,235'	Rush Creek junction	39.9	180.9	Inyo NF: Rush Creek, Silver Lake	June Lake	228
Rush Creek	7.0	+600', -3,250'	7,235'	Thousand Island Lake junction	43.0	177.8	Inyo NF: Rush Creek, Silver Lake	June Lake	228
River Trail	6.4	+360', -1,750'	8,300'	Garnet Lake junction	45.4	175.4	Inyo NF: River Trail, Agnew Meadow	Mammoth Lakes	229
Shadow Creek	4.5	+360', -840'	8,300'	Shadow Lake junction	49.0	171.8	Inyo NF: Shadow Creek, Agnew Meadow	Mammoth Lakes	229
Devils Postpile	0.75 (N), 0.6 (S)	+135', -25' (N); +160', -25' (S)	7,560'	northern (or southern) Devils Postpile junction	56.8 (57.5)	164.0 (163.3)	Inyo NF: JMT/PCT South Trailhead heading south; JMT/PCT North Trailhead heading north	Mammoth Lakes, Devils Postpile	230
Red's Meadow Resort to JMT**	0.3	+80', -0'	7,710'	western (or eastern) Reds Meadow junction	59.2 (59.3)	161.6 (161.5)	Inyo NF: JMT/PCT South Trailhead heading south; JMT/PCT North Trailhead heading north	Mammoth Lakes, Red's Meadow Resort	230
Mammoth Pass from Crater Meadow	3.2	+710', -370'	8,995'	lower Crater Meadow junction (Mammoth Pass)	62.0	158.8	Inyo NF: Red Cones, Mammoth Pass Trailhead	Mammoth Lakes	231
Duck Pass	5.6	+610', -1,670'	9,120'	Duck Pass junction	70.5	150.3	Inyo NF: Duck Lake Trailhead	Mammoth Lakes	231
McGee Pass	13.6	+2,780', -4,450'	7,870'	Tully Hole (McGee Pass junction)	76.8	144.0	Inyo NF: McGee Creek Trailhead	Mammoth Lakes	232

TRAIL	TRAIL LENGTH	ELEVATION GAIN/LOSS	TRAILHEAD ELEVATION	JMT JUNCTION	N-S	S-N	PERMITS	TOWNS ACCESSED	PAGE
Fish Creek Trail and Iva Bell Hot Springs	18.4	+2,065', -3,710'	9,200'	Cascade Valley (Fish Creek) junction	77.9	142.9	Inyo NF: Fish Creek Trail	Mammoth Lakes, Red's Meadow Resort	233
Goodale Pass	10.1	+690', -3,310'	7,825'	Goodale Pass junction	80.5	140.3	Sierra NF: Mono Creek Trail	Lake Thomas Edison, Vermilion Valley Resort (VVR)	233
Mono Pass	15.3	+4,200', -2,340'	10,220'	Mono Creek junction	86.6	134.2	Inyo NF: Mono Pass, Rock Creek	Mammoth Lakes, Bishop	234
Lake Edison**	1.5 (to ferry) 5.8 (to TH)	+550', -660' (TH)	7,825'	Lake Edison (Quail Meadows) junction	88.0	132.8	Sierra NF: Mono Creek Trail	Lake Thomas Edison, VVR	235
Bear Ridge	4.9	+100', -2,400'	7,735'	Bear Ridge junction	92.6	128.2	Sierra NF: Bear Ridge	Lake Thomas Edison, VVR	236
Bear Creek Cutoff	9.3	+1,030', -2,430'	7,560'	Bear Creek junction	94.8	126.0	Sierra NF: Bear Diversion	Lake Thomas Edison, VVR	236
Bear Creek Diversion Dam	8.9	+400', -2,340'	7,020'	Bear Creek junction	94.8	126.0	Sierra NF: Bear Diversion	Lake Thomas Edison, Mono Hot Springs, VVR	236
Florence Lake**	4.2 (to ferry) 7.7 (to TH)	+250', -720' (to ferry); +630', -1,075' (to TH)	7,330' (ferry) 7,350' (TH)	northern (or southern) Muir Trail Ranch cutoff	107.9 (109.7)	112.9 (111.1)	Sierra NF: Florence	Florence Lake, Muir Trail Ranch	237
Pine Creek Pass	17.8	+3,240', -4,000'	7,420'	Piute Creek junction	111.5	109.3	Inyo NF: Pine Creek Pass	Bishop	238
Piute Pass	17.1	+3,620', -2,410'	9,260'	Piute Creek junction	111.5	109.3	Inyo NF: Piute Pass, North Lake	Bishop	238
Bishop Pass	12.0	+3,370', -2,295'	9,795'	Bishop Pass junction	136.9	83.9	Inyo NF: Bishop Pass	Bishop	239
Taboose Pass	9.6	+810', -6,160'	5,430'	Taboose Pass junction	157.8	63	Inyo NF: Taboose Pass	Big Pine, Independence	239

TRAIL	TRAIL LENGTH	ELEVATION GAIN/LOSS	TRAILHEAD ELEVATION	JMT JUNCTION	N-S	S-N	PERMITS	TOWNS ACCESSED	PAGE
Sawmill Pass	12.5	+1,200', -6,960'	4,595'	Sawmill Pass junction	164.8	56	Inyo NF: Sawmill Pass	Big Pine, Independence	240
Woods Creek	13.5	+110', -3,560'	5,036'	Woods Creek junction	167.7	53.1	SEKI: Woods Creek	Cedar Grove (Kings Canyon NP)	241
Baxter Pass	10.4	+2,190', -6,310'	6,040'	Baxter Pass junction	172.4	48.4	Inyo NF: Baxter Pass	Independence	242
Kearsarge Pass (from north)**	7.4	+1,110', -2,560'	9,185'	Kearsarge Pass (or Charlotte Lake) junction	179.4 (179.6)	41.4 (41.2)	Inyo NF: Kearsarge Pass	Independence	242
Kearsarge Pass (from south)**	7.2	+1,345', -2,540'	9,185'	Bullfrog Lake junction	180	40.8	Inyo NF: Kearsarge Pass	Independence	243
Bubbs Creek	12.4	+0', -4,520'	5,036'	Bubbs Creek junction (Lower Vidette Meadow)	181.2	39.6	SEKI: Bubbs Creek	Cedar Grove (Kings Canyon NP)	243
Shepherd Pass	13.2	+1,755', -6,345'	6,300'	Shepherd Pass junction	194.3	26.5	Inyo NF: Shepherd Pass	Independence	244
New Army Pass, Cottonwood Lakes*	22.5	+4,080', -3,110'	10,060'	Pacific Crest Trail junction west of Crabtree Meadows	202.1	18.7	Inyo NF: Cottonwood Lakes	Lone Pine	245
Cottonwood Pass*	20.4	+3,580', -2,750'	9,940'	Pacific Crest Trail junction west of Crabtree Meadows	202.1	18.7	Inyo NF: Cottonwood Pass	Lone Pine	245

*Alternative starting point
**Common resupply point
North-to-south distances are in miles from Happy Isles, while south-to-north distances are in miles from Whitney Portal.
Elevation gain/loss is calculated from the JMT to the trailhead.

(Continued from page 223)

The Hike: 5.5 miles. From the Panorama Trail junction, head up switchbacks to a second junction. Turn right onto the Panorama Trail, which parallels the JMT west but is high above it, and enjoy beautiful vistas north. The trail descends to cross Illilouette Creek on a footbridge and then climbs steadily to Glacier Point. At a trail junction, stay right, and you will shortly reach Glacier Point.

Maps: USGS *Half Dome;* TH *Yosemite High Country*

Tuolumne Meadows, from Cathedral Lakes (section 2)

Access to: Tuolumne Meadows at Cathedral Lakes Trailhead (11S 290501E 4194217N)

Note: This trailhead is only available for hikers headed toward Yosemite Valley; if you're headed south, you need a permit for Lyell Canyon.

Trailhead Amenities: Only food-storage boxes at actual trailhead; water, toilets, visitor center, store, small café, campground, and buses to Yosemite Valley or Mammoth Lakes from Tuolumne Meadows

Getting to the Trailhead: The trailhead is near the western end of Tuolumne Meadows. Take CA 120 to Tuolumne Meadows, driving 20.5 miles west of Lee Vining or 38 miles east of Crane Flat (in Yosemite). Parking is available along the side of the road. See the map on page 21 for the layout of Tuolumne Meadows.

The Hike: 0.1 mile. From an X-junction, where the JMT turns right (east), head a short distance south (straight) from the JMT to reach the Cathedral Lakes Trailhead.

Maps: USGS *Tenaya Lake, Tioga Pass,* and *Vogelsang Peak;* TH *Yosemite High Country*

Tuolumne Meadows, from Lyell Canyon (section 2)

Access to: Tuolumne Meadows at wilderness permit parking area (11S 293760E 4194562N)

Trailhead Amenities: Water, toilets, visitor center, store, small café, campground, and buses to Yosemite Valley or Mammoth Lakes from Tuolumne Meadows

Getting to the Trailhead: The trailhead is near the eastern side of Tuolumne Meadows. Take CA 120 to Tuolumne Meadows, driving 18.3 miles west of Lee Vining or 40.2 miles east of Crane Flat (in Yosemite). Turn south at a signed turnoff for Tuolumne Lodge and almost immediately take a hard right onto a spur and into the backpacker's parking lot. See the map on page 21 for the layout of Tuolumne Meadows.

The Hike: None, as the JMT passes just south of the Tuolumne Meadows permit station.

Maps: USGS *Tenaya Lake, Tioga Pass,* and *Vogelsang Peak*; TH *Yosemite High Country*

Rush Creek Trail via Waugh Lake (section 3)

Access to: Rush Creek Trailhead near June Lake (11S 312679E 4183712N)

Trailhead Amenities: Toilets, campground, and Silver Lake Resort; the Yosemite Area Regional Transportation System (YARTS) bus between Yosemite and Mammoth Lakes stops at this trailhead each morning

Getting to the Trailhead: From the southern junction of US 395 and CA 158, drive southwest for 7.3 miles through June Lake Village, past June Mountain Ski Area, and just past Silver Lake Resort, to a large parking lot west of the road.

The Hike: 9.0 miles. Crossing the creek that descends from Davis Lake on a log, the trail climbs briefly, descends to cross Rush Creek on a wood bridge, and then skirts the north shore of Waugh Lake (with a few campsites), alternating between forest cover and dry slopes. Beyond you follow the moist terrain along the banks of Rush Creek (with several campsites), before detouring north around Gem Lake. Passing yet more campsites, you stay right at a junction to Gem Pass, and continue through mostly open, dry terrain as you leave Gem Lake and descend more steeply, first to Agnew Lake and then the Rush Creek Trailhead.

Maps: USGS *Mt. Ritter* and *Koip Peak*; TH *Mammoth High Country*

Rush Creek Trailhead from Thousand Island Lake (section 3)

Access to: Rush Creek Trailhead near June Lake (11S 312679E 4183712N)

Trailhead Amenities: Toilets, campground, and Silver Lake Resort; the YARTS bus between Yosemite and Mammoth Lakes stops at this trailhead each morning

Getting to the Trailhead: From the southern junction of US 395 and CA 158, drive southwest for 7.3 miles through June Lake Village, past June Mountain Ski Area, and just past Silver Lake Resort, to a large parking lot west of the road.

The Hike: 7.0 miles. From the junction at Thousand Island Lake, head east, staying left at a junction with the River Trail (after 1.0 mile). Stay left again at a junction 0.2 mile later; bearing right would lead to Agnew Pass (and eventually the Rush Creek Trailhead by a slightly longer route). Climbing steeply you reach Clark Lakes (and good campsites). Cross the Clark Lakes outlet stream and then bear left, climbing to a small lake with additional campsites. Now descend steeply, first through forest and later across a talus slope, to reach Agnew Lake. Cross the creek downstream of the dam and climb briefly to meet the main trail. A long, open, descending traverse takes you to the Rush Creek Trailhead.

Maps: USGS *Mt. Ritter* and *Koip Peak*; TH *Mammoth High Country*

Shadow Lake Trail to Agnew Meadows (section 4)

Access to: Agnew Meadows shuttle bus near Mammoth Lakes (11S 316610E 4172285N)

Trailhead Amenities: Toilets, water (currently at stables), nearby campgrounds, and shuttle bus to Mammoth Lakes

Getting to the Trailhead: At the junction of US 395 and CA 203, drive west for 3.8 miles through the town of Mammoth Lakes to the intersection where CA 203 turns right, toward Mammoth Mountain Ski Area and Devils Postpile. Turn right and drive 4.2 miles to the main Mammoth Mountain Ski Area. Between 7 a.m. and 7:30 p.m., mid-June–September, you are obliged to park here and take a shuttle bus to the Devils Postpile region, including Agnew Meadows; the buses run every 20 minutes. Before 7 a.m. and after 7:30 p.m., you may drive your own car, in which case you continue another 4.1 miles up and over Minaret Summit and down to the Agnew Meadows Trailhead, located at the first hairpin turn. Once on the spur road, keep left to reach the trailhead. The shuttle drops you on the main road at the hairpin turn, adding the 0.4-mile walk along the spur road to your journey. The shuttle bus fee is $7 per round-trip ticket, while descending in your own vehicle costs $10 per car. See **nps.gov/depo** for additional information.

The Hike: 4.5 miles. From the junction, the trail skirts the northern shore of Shadow Lake and then switchbacks down a steep slope to the Middle Fork of the San Joaquin River, where you turn right (south) onto the River Trail. You follow the River Trail for 0.9 mile, passing Olaine Lake and several campsites, and then trend left to climb out of the canyon and along a flat forest trail to Agnew Meadows. If you plan to take the shuttle bus, walk an additional 0.4 mile along the dirt road to reach the paved Minaret Summit Road—a distance included in the total above. Note that you can also leave the JMT at Garnet Lake, descending steeply to the River Trail. Cross the Middle Fork of the San Joaquin River as soon as you reach it—a fisherman's trail follows the western riverbank, but you want to be on the east side. The River Trail merges with the route to Shadow Lake at the junction north of Olaine Lake. The distance from Garnet Lake to Agnew Meadows for this variation is 6.4 miles and is the most direct way to exit from Garnet Lake.

Maps: USGS *Mt. Ritter* and *Mammoth Mtn.*; TH *Mammoth High Country*

Devils Postpile (section 4)

Access to: Devils Postpile Ranger Station near Mammoth Lakes (11S 316127E 4166584N)

Trailhead Amenities: Toilets, water, campground, visitor center, several nearby campgrounds, and shuttle bus to Mammoth Lakes

Getting to the Trailhead: Follow the directions to Agnew Meadows (page 229) as far as the hairpin turn; continue along Minaret Summit Road (the paved road) to the signed turnoff for Devils Postpile and descend briefly to reach a parking area. The distance from the Mammoth Mountain Ski Area parking lot is 8.1 miles. The shuttle service serving the Agnew Meadows Trailhead stops at Devils Postpile as well.

The Hike: 0.75 mile (from the north); 0.6 mile (from the south). From the northern X-junction, go southeast along the Middle Fork of San Joaquin River, bearing left at a junction, and immediately cross the river on a bridge just upstream of the postpiles. At the next junction head left, turning north and walking a short distance to the visitor center and a stop for seasonal shuttle bus service to Mammoth Mountain Ski Area. From the southern X-junction, head northeast, following the riverbank upstream to the bridge crossing.

Maps: USGS *Mammoth Mtn.*; TH *Mammoth High Country*; see also map on page 104

Red's Meadow Resort (section 4)

Access to: Red's Meadow Resort near Mammoth Lakes (11S 316934E 164899N)

Trailhead Amenities: Toilet, water, Red's Meadow Resort (seasonal lodging, café, store, pay showers), and campgrounds nearby, including Reds Meadow Campground

Getting to the Trailhead: Follow the directions on page 229 to Agnew Meadows as far as the hairpin turn. Continue on Minaret Summit Road (the paved road) to the signed turnoff for Red's Meadow Resort, nearly at the end of the road. At the very end, take a left turn to climb a hill to the resort; a right turn would lead down a dirt road to a parking lot for Rainbow Falls. The total distance from the Mammoth Mountain Ski Area parking lot is 9.6 miles.

The Hike: 0.3 mile from west Reds Meadow junction; 0.35 mile from eastern Reds Meadow junction. From either junction along the JMT, follow a spur trail north a short distance to reach the Red's Meadow Resort and a stop for seasonal shuttle bus service to Mammoth Mountain Ski Area.

Maps: USGS *Crystal Crag*; TH *Mammoth High Country*; see also map on page 104

Mammoth Pass Trail from Crater Meadow (Red Cones) to Horseshoe Lake (section 4)

Access to: Horseshoe Lake in Mammoth Lakes Basin (11S 321674E 4164596N)

Trailhead Amenities: Toilets, free summer shuttle service to the town of Mammoth Lakes (with all amenities), nearby campgrounds

Getting to the Trailhead: At the junction of US 395 and CA 203, drive west for 3.8 miles through the town of Mammoth Lakes to the intersection where CA 203 turns right, toward Mammoth Mountain Ski Resort and Devils Postpile. Continue straight, now on Lake Mary Road, and follow it past a turnoff to Twin Lakes and the Mammoth Pack Station. At a T-junction, head straight ahead around Lake Mary's north shore, and head toward Lake Mamie and Horseshoe Lake. Continue straight all the way to the road's end at Horseshoe Lake, about 5.7 miles past the junction to the Mammoth Mountain Ski Area. A free summer shuttle is available from The Village in Mammoth Lakes.

The Hike: 3.2 miles. Head east across Crater Meadow (many camping options) to reach a T-junction after 0.4 mile. Turn left (north) and then right (east) after another 0.1 mile. Now climb through forest to reach the trail from Upper Crater Meadow. Turn left (north) to climb gently over forested Mammoth Pass (9,350'), and then descend to McCleod Lake. Continue straight (east) at a junction at the east end of the lake, and you will shortly reach the trailhead at Horseshoe Lake. You can also reach the Horseshoe Lake Trailhead from the Upper Crater Meadow junction. This 4.3-mile hike heads east from the JMT and also immediately reaches a junction where you head right (east), walking through forest to reach the previously described route a little west of Mammoth Pass (after 2.3 miles).

Maps: USGS *Crystal Crag*; TH *Mammoth High Country*

Duck Pass Trail (section 5)

Access to: Mammoth Lakes Basin; Coldwater Campground/Duck Pass Trailhead (11S 324448E 4162143N)

Trailhead Amenities: Toilets, water, and campground. You are in a lake basin southwest of Mammoth Lakes, and there are campgrounds, lodging, and a few stores widely scattered along the roads through the basin. A free summer shuttle to the town of Mammoth Lakes stops at the Lake Mary store, 0.7 mile down the road from the trailhead.

Getting to the Trailhead: At the junction of US 395 and CA 203, drive west for 3.8 miles through the town of Mammoth Lakes to the intersection where CA 203 turns right, toward Mammoth Mountain Ski Area and Devils Postpile. Continue straight, now on Lake Mary

Road, and follow it past a turnoff to Twin Lakes and the Mammoth Pack Station. At a T-junction, turn left to skirt Lake Mary's eastern shore. At a second T-junction, past Pine City Campground, turn left into Coldwater Campground and follow signs to a large parking lot at the top of Coldwater Campground, 5.2 miles past the junction to the Mammoth Mountain Ski Area. The Duck Pass Trail begins behind the toilets. Do not take the spur trail that immediately heads up and right toward Emerald Lake.

The Hike: 5.6 miles. From the Duck Pass junction climb up through rocky terrain with scattered trees to reach Duck Lake. Camping is not allowed within 300 feet of Duck Lake's outlet. Skirt the western edge of the lake, passing a junction to Pika Lake (and camping), before reaching Duck Pass, 10,797 feet. Descend tight switchbacks on the north-facing slope, which can hold snow well into July, and reach Barney Lake. Continue down, passing multiple lakes, each with campsites, to reach the trailhead.

Maps: USGS *Bloody Mtn.*; TH *Mammoth High Country*

McGee Pass Trail (section 5)

Access to: Crowley Lake region, 8 miles south of Mammoth Lakes on US 395; McGee Pass Trailhead (11S 340819E 4157324N)

Trailhead Amenities: Toilet, nearby campground, and pack station down the road. There is no public transit from (or near to) this trailhead, but it is a high-use trail.

Getting to the Trailhead: From US 395, 8.2 miles south of Mammoth (or 30.5 miles north of Bishop), turn southwest on signed McGee Canyon Road and follow it 3.3 miles past McGee Pack Station to a road-end parking loop.

The Hike: 13.6 miles. Follow Fish Creek upstream from Tully Hole, initially on the south bank, crossing after 0.9 mile. Continue up through meadows and forest, with many camping options until about 10,400 feet. The trail then climbs more steeply to the top of McGee Pass, switchbacking among clumps of whitebark pines (with small bivvy sites). The eastern side of McGee Pass holds snow late, and you descend a broad slope before trending south and descending metamorphic talus to Little McGee Lake. The trail continues down McGee Creek among meadows and past many trickles (and more camping options) to reach first a little-used junction leading to the Scheelore Mine (stay right) and just thereafter a second junction where you head left to the McGee Pass Trailhead (right takes you to Steelhead Lake). Continue down McGee Creek, crossing once on a sturdy bridge and lower on a second bridge.

Maps: USGS *Bloody Mtn., Graveyard Peak, Mt. Abbott,* and *Convict Lake;* TH *Mammoth High Country* and *Mono Divide High Country*

Fish Creek Trail and Iva Bell Hot Springs (sections 4 and 5)

Access to: Red's Meadow Resort near Mammoth Lakes (11S 316934E 164899N)

Trailhead Amenities: Toilet, water, Red's Meadow Resort (seasonal lodging, café, store, pay showers), and campgrounds nearby, including Reds Meadow Campground.

Getting to the Trailhead: See the description for Red's Meadow Resort on page 230.

The Hike: 18.4 miles. The hike down Cascade Valley is mostly through forest, but in stretches you are treated to the creek tumbling over slabs; there are campsites throughout the descent. Before long you come to a crossing of Fish Creek; search upstream for a log on which to cross. Continuing down, alongside marshy meadows and through forest, remain straight at a right junction to Purple Lake and a left junction where the trail crosses Fish Creek and climbs up the south side of the canyon. The descent continues, crossing Fish Creek again (this time on a bridge), shortly before you descend to Iva Bell Hot Springs (8.0 miles from the JMT), a collection of warm pools with many nearby campsites. The trail now descends into Fish Valley, at the western end of which is another creek crossing on a bridge. The trail now switchbacks up a dry slope and slowly bends northward into the Middle Fork of the San Joaquin drainage. You follow Crater Creek for several miles, before a descending traverse takes you toward Rainbow Falls. Here you join a popular day hike and continue north to the Red's Meadow Resort. *Note:* It is a beautiful walk along Fish Creek, but if you are in a hurry to exit the JMT, it is shorter to walk north along the JMT and exit at Duck Pass. An intermediate choice is to follow Fish Creek to the Purple Lake junction and then climb back to the JMT to reach Duck Pass.

Maps: USGS *Crystal Crag, Graveyard Peak,* and *Sharktooth Peak*; TH *Mammoth High Country* and *Mono Divide High Country*

Goodale Pass (sections 5 and 6)

Access to: Lake Thomas Edison, Vermilion Valley Resort, Mono Hot Springs; Lake Edison Trailhead (11S 322091E 4138859N)

Trailhead Amenities: Campground, water, and toilets; Vermilion Valley Resort 0.5 mile to south. There is no public transit to this location, but VVR has Internet access, and some cell phones have service near the shores of Lake Edison, should you need to arrange for a pickup.

Getting to the Trailhead: From Fresno, take CA 168 northeast through Clovis and up into the foothills, through the community of Shaver Lake. Continue straight at a turnoff to Huntington Lake, and reach a T-junction near the community of Lakeshore, 67.4 miles from CA

180. Turn right (east) onto Huntington Lake/Kaiser Pass Road, which soon becomes narrow and twisting. At Kaiser Pass, it becomes even more narrow and twisting before descending past the High Sierra Ranger Station to a Y-junction, 15.1 miles from Huntington Lake. A left turn here heads to Mono Hot Springs Resort, Lake Edison, and Vermilion Valley Resort, and a right turn goes to Florence Lake. Take a left. You next pass turnoffs first to Mono Hot Springs (on your left) and then parking areas for the Bear Creek Cutoff and Bear Ridge Trails (on your right). Cross beneath the Lake Edison Dam, and pass a junction for the Vermilion Valley Resort. Now on a dirt road, continue straight, passing turnoffs to the main Vermilion Campground (on your right), the pack station (on your left), and finally follow signs right to the Lake Edison Trailhead, a distance of 8.3 miles from the Y-junction. This very slow drive takes 2.5–3 hours from Fresno.

The Hike: 10.1 miles. The trail trends west, descending to cross the Papoose Lake outlet, and then stays left at a junction and climbs toward Goodale Pass. The trail climbs steeply, reaching a second junction in a sandy flat; again stay left and continue the climb to Goodale Pass, a sandy notch in a landscape of rocky outcrops. The trail switchbacks down a steep slope to reach Cold Creek and several long meadows (with camping options). Descending farther, you cross the creek and reach Graveyard Meadows and then a junction where you stay left. The trail now descends the steep slope overlooking Lake Edison before merging with the Lake Edison Trail and turning westward. Just beyond, stay right at a junction to reach a bridge over Cold Creek, before soon reaching the Lake Edison Trailhead. Vermilion Valley Resort is 0.5 mile south of the trailhead. Either follow a sometimes-marked use trail south and west from the trailhead, or follow the road first west and then south.

Maps: USGS *Graveyard Peak* and *Sharktooth Peak*; TH *Mono Divide High Country*

Mono Pass Trail (section 6)

Access to: Mosquito Flat Trailhead (11S 345477E 4144341N) and beyond to Toms Place, 24 miles north of Bishop and 15 miles south of Mammoth Lakes on US 395

Trailhead Amenities: Toilets and, down Rock Creek Road, campgrounds, lodging, cafés, and stores. There is no public transit from (or near to) this trailhead, but it is a high-use trail. The Eastern Sierra Transit buses stop at Toms Place.

Getting to the Trailhead: From US 395 at Toms Place, turn west on Rock Creek Road and follow the road past Rock Creek Lake. Beyond the turnoff for the lake, the road becomes one lane. Continue all the way to the road-end parking lot, 9.2 miles from US 395.

The Hike: 15.3 miles. Leaving the JMT, climb over a shallow ridge and descend into the Mono Creek drainage. Follow the drainage up, passing through beautiful forests, crossing multiple side creeks, and staring at the steep granite walls of the Mono Recesses to the south. There are camping options at most locations along the creek. The trail climbs steadily but gently until you approach the Pioneer Basin junctions. You now climb more steadily, passing Trail Lake (lovely campsites), reaching Summit Lake (alpine camping options), and then Mono Pass, 11.9 miles from the JMT. You now descend a sandy and rocky gully and then switchback down a long, dry slope above Ruby Lake. The last campsites are at Ruby Lake, before you continue your descent to the Mosquito Flat Trailhead.

Maps: USGS *Graveyard Peak*, *Mt. Abbott*, and *Mt. Morgan*; TH *Mono Divide High Country*

Lake Edison Trail (section 6)

Access to: Lake Thomas Edison, Vermilion Valley Resort, Mono Hot Springs; Lake Edison Trailhead (11S 322091E 4138859N)

Trailhead Amenities: Campground, water, and toilets; Vermilion Valley Resort 0.5 mile to south. There is no public transit to this location, but VVR has Internet access, and some cell phones have service near the shores of Lake Edison, should you need to arrange for a pickup.

Getting to the Trailhead: See the description for Goodale Pass on page 233.

The Hike: 1.5 miles to ferry or 5.8 miles to the Lake Edison Trailhead. Heading west, the route passes Quail Meadows, with marshy stretches of trail and spectacular wildflowers. Continuing through forest, after 1.3 miles you reach a junction, with left (south) signposted for the ferry wharf (and campsites) and straight (west) leading around Lake Edison. The spur trail to the wharf is just over 0.1 mile, though if water levels are low, you might have to walk approximately 1 mile across the dry reservoir bed to reach a makeshift ferry landing. (See page 24 for more information on the Edison ferry.) Meanwhile, the main trail circles around the lake, mostly on dry scrubby slopes, with just a few camping options near the beginning. Soon after the Goodale Pass Trail merges from the right, the trail bends rights (north) to cross Cold Creek on a large bridge. Stay right again at the junction for the pack station, and soon reach the Lake Edison Trailhead. Vermilion Valley Resort is 0.5 mile south of the trailhead. Either follow a sometimes-marked use trail south and west from the trailhead, or follow the road first west and then south.

Maps: USGS *Graveyard Peak* and *Sharktooth Peak*; TH *Mono Divide High Country*

Bear Ridge Trail (section 6)

Access to: Lake Thomas Edison, Vermilion Valley Resort, Mono Hot Springs; Bear Ridge Trailhead near Lake Edison Dam (11S 324706E 4137456N)

Trailhead Amenities: Toilets and, nearby, Vermilion Valley Resort (on the north side of the dam) and several campgrounds. There is no public transit to this location, but VVR has Internet access, and some cell phones have service near the shores of Lake Edison, should you need to arrange for a pickup.

Getting to the Trailhead: Refer to the driving directions to Goodale Pass on page 233. However, just as you approach the dam across Lake Edison, turn right into the signposted parking lot.

The Hike: 4.9 miles. This trail descends the north side of Bear Ridge, descending steadily at first through open forest and later traversing moister stretches of forest (with possible, but little-used camping). Beyond, the trail traverses drier slopes high above the unseen Lake Edison. The lake only comes into view along the final descent to the trailhead.

Maps: USGS *Florence Lake* and *Graveyard Peak*; TH *Mono Divide High Country*; see map on pages 124–125 for additional information

Bear Creek Trail (section 6)

Access to: Lake Thomas Edison, Vermilion Valley Resort, Mono Hot Springs; Bear Creek Cutoff Trailhead (11S 324269E 4136674N); Bear Creek Diversion Dam Trailhead (11S 322527E 4134085N)

Trailhead Amenities: None, but nearby are Vermilion Valley Resort (on the north side of the dam; the closest facilities if you follow the cutoff trail), Mono Hot Springs Resort (including a post office; the closest facilities if you walk to the Diversion Dam), and several campgrounds. There is no public transit to this location, but VVR has Internet access, and some cell phones have service near the shores of Lake Edison, should you need to arrange for a pickup.

Getting to this Trailhead: Refer to the driving directions to Lake Edison (Goodale Pass) on page 233 as far as the Y-junction. Turn left at the Y-junction, and after 2.5 miles reach the Bear Diversion Dam Road junction (with an off-highway vehicle route) on your right. Passenger cars can't go beyond here nor can less robust four-wheel-drive vehicles, so the trail description starts from this point. Continue another 2.8 miles along the main road to reach the Bear Creek Cutoff Trailhead, again on your right.

The Hike: 8.9 miles (Bear Diversion Dam) or 9.3 miles (Bear Creek Cutoff). Though there are two possible exits, both trails begin by following Bear Creek west. The first 0.7 mile is along Bear Creek, with multiple campsites. The trail then diverges and climbs over a dry slab ridge, dotted with junipers. Descending gradually, the trail doesn't again intersect Bear Creek until 3.1 miles from the JMT. You now follow a beautiful stretch of creek with cascades, deep swimming pools, and campsites where the valley floor is wide and flat enough. After just over 6 miles you reach an unmarked trail junction, beyond a glade of aspens and where the landscape suddenly lacks trees (11S 325805E 4134581N). Straight ahead continues to the Bear Diversion Dam, while right (north) is the Bear Creek Cutoff that crosses Bear Ridge. The route to the Bear Diversion Dam is marginally shorter and all downhill, but you exit much farther from Vermilion Valley Resort. To reach the Bear Diversion Dam, continue straight, passing a trailhead sign after 0.7 mile. You are now on a rugged off-highway vehicle road and follow it for 2.1 miles to the paved road. If you choose to follow the Bear Creek Cutoff, climb switchbacks up a dry slope of scrubs and then descend the north side of Bear Ridge to the trailhead.

Maps: USGS *Florence Lake* and *Mt. Givens*; TH *Mono Divide High Country*; see map on pages 124–125 for additional information

Florence Lake Trail past Muir Trail Ranch (section 7)

Access to: Muir Trail Ranch (11S 333197E 4122683N); Florence Lake ferry wharf (11S 327911E 4124218N); Florence Lake Trailhead (11S 325027 4126806N)

Trailhead Amenities: Toilets, water, and Florence Lake Store; the Florence Lake ferry runs five times daily across the lake.

Getting to the Trailhead: Follow the directions under the Lake Edison Trail description (see Goodale Pass on page 233) as far as the Y-junction at the base of Kaiser Pass, but then turn right and follow the road 6.4 miles to its end at Florence Lake.

The Hike: 4.2 miles (Florence ferry) or 7.7 miles (Florence Trailhead). The following description and mileages begin at the trail junction between the two JMT cutoffs, a short distance east of the Muir Trail Ranch. From this point, instead of heading left (south) to the ranch, stay straight (west), signposted for Florence Lake. The trail is nearly flat as it crosses Blayney Meadows (with camping options), but then climbs slightly up a slope to Double Meadow, before slowly descending a dry slope to a junction. Here the right fork leads 0.5 mile to the ferry wharf, while the main trail continues southwest to cross the South Fork of the San Joaquin on a bridge (with campsites nearby). The trail around Florence Lake traverses the south side of the lake, with several short ascents and descents around steep bluffs.

Maps: USGS *Florence Lake* and *Ward Mountain*; TH *Mono Divide High Country*

Pine Creek Pass Trail (section 7)

Access to: US 395, 10 miles north of Bishop; Pine Creek Trailhead (11S 350320E 4136107N)

Trailhead Amenities: Toilets and pack station. There is no public transit to this trailhead, but on most days there is sufficient traffic that you will be able to find a lift to Bishop.

Getting to the Trailhead: From the junction of Line Street and Main Street in Bishop, head north on US 395 for 10.7 miles to the signed road to Rovana. Follow this road 9.4 miles west to a signed parking area on your left (south).

The Hike: 17.8 miles. This long but beautiful hike begins with a climb up the narrow, rocky Piute Canyon: both sides of the canyon have tall, steep cliffs. After 2.5 miles the canyon becomes less steep and broader, permitting occasional camping, but still climbs steadily to Hutchinson Meadow (5.1 miles from JMT). Here you head left toward Pine Creek Pass and climb gently but steadily up French Canyon. The valley floor consists of a succession of meadows—some wetter, others drier, but all beautiful. A special treat is a waterfall draining from the Royce Lakes (on the north side). At a junction, head left and then climb more steeply to Pine Creek Pass (11,100'), which lies between two small lakes; camping is nearby. Now begins the long descent, mostly along creeks and through small meadows until you reach a junction between Honeymoon and Pine Creek Lakes (both with campsites). Turn right and descent through forest and along lakeshores until you pass Lower Pine Creek Lake (and more camping). Now the terrain steepens and the valley narrows as the trail descends steadily. Often rocky underfoot, this is a tiring descent, but you are rewarded with beautiful views. The final stretch of trail is once more near Pine Creek before you pass through the pack station and reach the parking lot.

Maps: USGS *Mt. Henry, Mt. Hilgard, Mt. Darwin*, and *Mt. Tom*; TH *Mono Divide High Country*

Piute Pass Trail (section 7)

Access to: Bishop; North Lake Trailhead (11S 355703E 4121119N)

Trailhead Amenities: Toilets, water, campground, and pack station. There is no public transport to this trailhead, but it is very popular, and you should have no difficulty finding a lift to Bishop.

Getting to the Trailhead: From the junction of US 395 and CA 168 (West Line Street) in Bishop, go southwest 18 miles and turn right onto a dirt road to North Lake (this is a mile after Aspendell). Drive 1.6 miles along the North Lake Road and then turn right to reach a backpacker's parking area next to the pack station (11S 356469E 4121476N). The trailhead is 0.5 mile ahead, in the North Lake

Campground, but there is no parking here (this final stretch of road is included in the hiking mileage).

The Hike: 17.1 miles. Follow the same path as the Pine Creek Pass hike for the first 5.1 miles to Hutchinson Meadow. The Piute Pass Trail then heads right (south) toward Piute Pass, continuing up first through forest (with campsites), later sections of slab, and finally moist alpine meadows. The preferred trail lies high above the wettest meadows and tarns, limiting damage, before passing an unsigned spur trail to Desolation Lake (and ample campsites), and then climbing the final slopes to the pass. Descending the east side the trail passes a sequence of tarns and lakes, separated by moist meadows. Campsites can be found throughout this stretch. Below Loch Leven Lake the terrain dries and steepens, as you pass the red Piute Crags on your descent to the trailhead. At the bottom turn left (north) toward the campground. Since there is no parking here, you must now walk 0.5 mile down the dirt road, turning left onto a signposted spur road. (This distance is included in the mileage.)

Maps: USGS *Mt. Henry, Mt. Hilgard, Mt. Darwin,* and *Mt. Tom;* TH *Mono Divide High Country*

Bishop Pass Trail (section 8)

Access to: Bishop; South Lake Trailhead (11S 361066E 4114607N)

Trailhead Amenities: Toilets and, nearby, pack station, campgrounds, and resorts. There is no public transport to this trailhead, but it is very popular, and you should have no difficulty finding a lift to Bishop.

Getting to the Trailhead: From the junction of US 395 and CA 168 (West Line Street) in Bishop, go southwest 15.0 miles to a junction. Turn left toward Bishop Lake and follow the road 7.1 miles to its end at a parking area at South Lake.

The Hike: 12.0 miles. The trail climbs diligently out of Le Conte Canyon, switchbacking up with little reprieve except the endless views and a few campsites, until reaching Dusy Basin. From Dusy Basin upward the landscape is gentler with beautiful lakes and many campsites. The trail, however, continues its upward trajectory, reaching the broad-topped Bishop Pass (11,972'). The descent of the east side takes you past lake after lake, each with camping choices and most with spectacular views.

Maps: USGS *North Palisade* and *Mt. Thompson;* TH *Kings Canyon High Country*

Taboose Pass Trail (section 9)

Access to: US 395, 12 miles south of Big Pine, 14 miles north of Independence; Taboose Pass Trailhead (11S 381987E 4096560N)

Trailhead Amenities: None. This trailhead receives little traffic, so if you haven't arranged a pickup or have a car at the trailhead, assume that you will also have to walk the 5.7 miles to US 395 before finding a lift.

Getting to the Trailhead: From US 395, drive 12.2 miles south of Big Pine (at the junction of Crocker Street) or 14.3 miles north of Independence (at the junction of Market Street). Turn west onto paved Aberdeen Station Road (signposted for Taboose Creek as well). After 1.2 miles go straight at a four-way junction with Tinemaha Road. Your road is now named Taboose Creek Road and becomes a narrow dirt road. After an additional 0.5 mile, bear right; you are still driving on the most prominent of the dirt road options. Stay right at a Y after 1.9 miles and continue straight to the trailhead, a total of 5.7 miles from US 395.

The Hike: 9.6 miles. The trail climbs gently up the southern slope of the broad valley draining from Taboose Pass. Once you have completed the initial climb through forest, you open into a landscape of meadows and sandy expanses, with scattered campsites. After 1.7 miles you intersect a second trail, the northern Taboose Trail, unmaintained and not signposted. The trail continues its gentle ascent to the pass (11,418'), crosses a stretch of beautiful tarns nestled between slabs, and begins a long descent of the east side. Between elevations of 9,700 and 8,300 feet, there are several campsites, with one option even lower. The descent is long—nearly 6,000 feet down—and often steep and with cobble on the upper sections, but at least the lower stretches of the trail are sandy and make for easy walking. Note that if you are coming from the north, it is considerably faster to take the abandoned northern Taboose Trail, which leaves the JMT at 11S 371662E 4092802N, but this trail is difficult to follow. Head straight to the creek and cross it; the trail becomes obvious once on the other bank. Some sections of this trail run through wet meadows, and you are asked to skirt those far to the north to avoid damaging the wetlands. The two trails merge 1.7 miles up the trail.

Maps: USGS *Mt. Pinchot* and *Aberdeen*; TH *Kings Canyon High Country*

Sawmill Pass Trail (section 10)

Access to: US 395, 18 miles south of Big Pine, 8.5 miles north of Independence; Sawmill Pass Trailhead (11S 385183E 4088677N)

Trailhead Amenities: None. This trailhead receives very little traffic, so if you haven't arranged a pickup or have a car at the trailhead, assume that you will also have to walk the 4.0 miles to US 395 before finding a lift.

Getting to the Trailhead: From US 395, 18.0 miles south of Big Pine (at the junction of Crocker Street) or 8.5 miles north of Independence (at the junction of Market Street), turn west onto the dirt Black Rock Springs Road. Go west 0.8 mile to a junction with paved Tinemaha Road. Turn right and continue for 1.2 miles. Then turn left onto Division Creek Road and follow it for 2.0 miles to the trailhead.

The Hike: 12.5 miles. After crossing a tributary to Woods Creek, the trail sidles up and across the western slope of Mt. Cedric Wright, before bending east and reaching the basin that holds Woods Lake and many smaller lakes. While sections of this trail have been recently rebuilt and sport well-constructed steps, stretches higher up are indistinct and require careful attention. Campsites exist at all the lakes. Continuing upward you reach the broad plateau, the southern end of which is Sawmill Pass (11,347'), and descend the steep eastern escarpment. Down, down go tight switchbacks, leading first to a tarn and then Sawmill Lake, with some campsites along the eastern shores. The descent continues to Sawmill Meadow (more camping) and then across to Hogsback Creek. Continuing down, and weaving through beautiful riparian vegetation, the trail eventually traverses across the Hogsback (even ascending slightly) before descending the eastern side of Sawmill Point on sandy switchbacks. The trail finally trends north, crossing several dry creeks before reaching the trailhead.

Maps: USGS *Mt. Pinchot* and *Aberdeen*; TH *Kings Canyon High Country*

Woods Creek Trail (section 10)

Access to: Roads End at Cedar Grove in Kings Canyon National Park (11S 358860E 4073060N)

Trailhead Amenities: Toilets, water, National Park Service ranger station, and, nearby, Cedar Grove (lodging, café, small store, and campgrounds). There is no public transit to this popular tourist location, making a private vehicle or private shuttle almost a necessity to reach the closest shuttle location, the Giant Forest in Sequoia National Park, or the closest train station, Fresno.

Getting to the Trailhead: Starting in Fresno at the intersection of CA 180 and CA 41, go east 53.6 miles to a T-junction just inside Kings Canyon National Park. Turn left (north) and drive an additional 35.7 miles, past Grant Grove Village, over a summit, and then down into Kings Canyon to the Roads End Trailhead, 6 miles east of Cedar Grove Village.

The Hike: 13.5 miles. This trail follows Woods Creek, descending steadily through Castle Dome Meadows to the eastern end of Paradise Valley and a large camping area with food-storage boxes. The trail is nearly flat along the long length of Paradise Valley, before dropping steeply again as it descends mostly dry scrubby slopes toward Kings Canyon below. At a large footbridge, you continue straight; the trail from the left is the Bubbs Creek Trail. Now follow the final 2 flat miles to Roads End, the trailhead.

Maps: USGS *Mt. Clarence King* and *The Sphinx*; TH *Kings Canyon High Country*

Baxter Pass Trail (section 10)

Access to: Independence; Baxter Pass Trailhead (11S 384385E 4078238N)

Trailhead Amenities: Campground nearby. This trailhead receives very little use, so if you haven't arranged a pickup or have a car at the trailhead, assume that you will also have to walk the 5.6 miles to US 395 before finding a lift.

Getting to the Trailhead: From Independence (at the junction of Market Street), head north on US 395 for 2.3 miles. Turn west onto paved Fish Hatchery Road and go 1.2 miles to a Y-junction. Go right here, passing Oak Creek Campground, to the trailhead, 4.4 miles from the Y-junction.

The Hike: 10.4 miles. From the junction at Dollar Lake, this little used trail traverses up and north across a talus slope and then cuts east into the Baxter Lakes Basin, where there are good campsites. It then bends south and climbs steep switchbacks to the broad summit of Baxter Pass (12,270'). The trail down the east side is steep and in places difficult to follow. You first descend a talus slope and then skirt through patches of alpine meadow and clumps of trees (with a few campsites), before beginning a long stretch along the north bank of the river. The trail is often overgrown here, but continue down until you find an obvious place to cross to the south bank. From here down the trail is obvious, passing beneath clumps of tall firs and elsewhere descending dry slopes. The trail crosses Oak Creek once more, about 1 mile before the trailhead.

Maps: USGS *Mt. Clarence King* and *Kearsarge Peak*; TH *Kings Canyon High Country*

Kearsarge Pass Trail, from North (section 11)

Access to: Onion Valley near Independence; Kearsarge Pass Trailhead (11S 380384E 4070278N)

Trailhead Amenities: Toilet, water, and campground. This is a popular trailhead for both day hikers and backpackers, and you should have no difficulty finding a ride to Independence.

Getting to the Trailhead: In Independence, turn west from US 395 onto Market Street (Onion Valley Road), and follow it for 12.5 steep, winding miles to a large parking area that serves three trailheads. Kearsarge Pass is the middle and most obvious trailhead.

The Hike: 7.4 miles. From either the northern Kearsarge Pass junction or the Charlotte Lake junction, head east; the two spurs join after just 0.3 mile. The trail climbs and then traverses the slope north of Bullfrog Lake and the Kearsarge Lakes, allowing for beautiful views to the south. Continue up and along, crossing a few small trickles, a spur trail that leads to the Kearsarge Lakes (and Bullfrog Lake), and eventually the sandy summit of Kearsarge Pass (11,810'). The trail makes several long, sweeping zigzags down the eastern escarpment, before reaching a steeper section with views to Heart Lake. A series of tighter switchbacks and additional descent brings you near the creek at the Flower Lake outlet (campsites at the lake). You continue down past Gilbert Lake and Little Pothole Lake, both with camping, before descending the final, mostly dry slope to the trailhead. Near the bottom, stay right at a junction; the left path leads to Golden Trout Lakes.

Maps: USGS *Mt. Clarence King* and *Kearsarge Peak*; TH *Kings Canyon High Country*

Kearsarge Pass Trail, from South (section 11)

Access to: Onion Valley near Independence; Kearsarge Pass Trailhead (11S 380384E 4070278N)

Trailhead Amenities: Toilet, water, and campground. This is a popular trailhead for both day hikers and backpackers, and you should have no difficulty finding a ride to Independence.

Getting to the Trailhead: Follow the directions to Kearsarge Pass Trail, from the north, on the previous page.

The Hike: 7.2 miles. From the Bullfrog Lake junction, climb gently, passing first a tarn and then Bullfrog Lake (no camping here). The trail then climbs past beautiful meadows, small stands of trees, and across a few trickles en route to the Kearsarge Lakes. An indistinct spur trail leads to the lakes and many campsites; they lie well south of the trail you are following. Eventually the trail makes a steep ascent on a dry, sandy slope, intersecting the main Kearsarge Pass Trail just west of the pass's summit. See the hike description above for the descent from Kearsarge Pass.

Maps: USGS *Mt. Clarence King* and *Kearsarge Peak*; TH *Kings Canyon High Country*

Bubbs Creek Trail (section 11)

Access to: Roads End at Cedar Grove in Kings Canyon National Park (11S 358860E 4073060N)

Trailhead Amenities: Toilets, water, National Park Service ranger station, and, nearby, Cedar Grove (with lodging, a café, a small store, and campgrounds). There is no public transit to this popular tourist location, making a private vehicle or shuttle almost a necessity to reach the closest shuttle location, the Giant Forest in Sequoia National Park, or the closest train station, Fresno.

Getting to the Trailhead: Follow the directions to Woods Creek Trail, on page 241.

The Hike: 12.4 miles. Once beyond Lower Vidette Meadow, the trail descends steadily, switchbacking down a dry slope to Junction Meadow (and a side trail to East Lake). A campsite with food-storage boxes is located at the western end of the meadow. The trail continues down, the canyon never steep and never flat, meandering in and out of forest versus drier, shorter vegetation. Another large camping area is near where Charlotte Creek flows across the trail. More miles down-canyon is a final camping area, near where the Sphinx Trail departs to the south. The trail now switchbacks down a steep scrubby slope overlooking Kings Canyon, while Bubbs Creek drops steeply in a gorge to your south. Suddenly you reach Kings Canyon and flat terrain. The trail crosses Woods Creek on a foot-bridge, and you walk the final flat 2 miles to the Roads End (Cedar Grove) Trailhead.

Maps: USGS *Mt. Clarence King* and *The Sphinx*; TH *Kings Canyon High Country* and *Mt. Whitney High Country*

Shepherd Pass Trail (section 12)

Access to: Shepherd Pass Trailhead near Independence (11S 385893E 4065164N)

Trailhead Amenities: None. This is a relatively low-use trail, and find-ing a ride to Independence is likely to be difficult.

Getting to the Trailhead: In Independence, turn from US 395 west onto Market Street (Onion Valley Road). Go 4.4 miles to Foothill Road, turn left, and go 1.3 miles to a Y-junction, where you stay right. Continue for an additional 2.0 miles and then turn right (west). Continue another 1.4 miles to the road's end, staying right where two less distinct dirt roads bear south.

The Hike: 13.2 miles. From the JMT, the trail climbs gradually to Shep-herd Pass, at first through a few stands of trees and then into open alpine tundra. The landscape here is moist with many trickles, and the trail has recently been rerouted to avoid most of them. The views west, south, and north are spectacular right up until you reach the sandy pass; now you stare down the steep eastern escarpment. You switchback down a steep slope, the trail in need of repair in places, before reaching gentler slopes and the Pothole and campsites. Con-tinued descent of gentler slopes brings you to Anvil Camp and then Mahogany Flat (with more camping). The trail soon makes an unwel-come ascent as it crosses from Shepherd Creek (which cliffs out lower down) into Symmes Creek. The switchbacks from the shoulder down to Symmes Creek are gentle and correspondingly long—perfect for a long climb but slow for the descent. The final mile of trail descends on the banks of Symmes Creek to reach the road; this stretch of trail was recently washed out and can be difficult to follow.

Maps: USGS *Mt. Williamson*; TH *Mt. Whitney High Country*

PCT South, from Crabtree to Cottonwood Lakes (section 12)

Access to: Lone Pine; Cottonwood Lakes Trailhead in Horseshoe Meadows (11S 395230E 4034656N)

Trailhead Amenities: Toilets, water, and campground. You will probably get a ride from this trailhead to Lone Pine, but you should arrange for a shuttle if you don't have several hours—or more—to spare.

Getting to the Trailhead: Turn west from US 395 in Lone Pine onto Whitney Portal Road. Go 3.1 miles and turn left onto Horseshoe Meadow Road. Go straight 19.2 miles and then turn right to the trailhead marked for Cottonwood Lakes and New Army Pass (not Cottonwood Pass). Follow this road 0.5 mile to the end. This is an alternative way to begin the JMT if you cannot get a permit to begin the hike out of Whitney Portal.

The Hike: 22.5 miles. At the Crabtree junction the JMT turns east to reach its terminus on Mt. Whitney, while you follow the route of the Pacific Crest Trail (PCT) south. You cross the open sandy country leading up Guyot Pass and then drop into Rock Creek. The trail now follows Rock Creek (passing the Rock Creek Ranger Station), staying left where the PCT heads south to Cottonwood Pass. Higher up, you skirt one small lake and almost reach a second before turning south to switchback up to a broad plateau and New Army Pass (12,310'), 13.7 miles from the JMT junction. (There is camping throughout the ascent of Rock Creek.) You now descend switchbacks to the Cottonwood Lakes Basin, picturesque and containing excellent campsites. As you leave the lakes, you cross Cottonwood Creek twice in rapid succession, pass the Golden Trout Camp, and continue through dry, quiet flat forest to the trailhead.

Maps: USGS *Mt. Whitney*, *Johnson Peak*, and *Cirque Lake*; TH *Mt. Whitney High Country*

PCT South, from Crabtree to Cottonwood Pass (section 12)

Access to: Lone Pine; Cottonwood Pass Trailhead in Horseshoe Meadows (11S 395166E 4034116N)

Trailhead Amenities: Toilets, water, and campground. You will probably get a ride from this trailhead to Lone Pine, but you should arrange for a shuttle if you don't have several hours—or more—to spare.

Getting to the Trailhead: Follow the directions for Cottonwood Lakes as far as a junction where you stay straight for Cottonwood Pass (not right to New Army Pass Trailhead), and follow this road to its end. This is an alternative way to begin the JMT if you cannot get a permit to begin the hike out of Whitney Portal.

The Hike: 20.4 miles. Follow the description for Cottonwood Lakes as far as Rock Creek. As you are ascending Rock Creek, continue along the Pacific Crest Trail (PCT) where it bears right (south) and climbs out of the river drainage. The trail climbs through scattered trees and across sandy flats above Siberian Outpost and then to the west of Cirque Peak as it continues south. You descend into the little basin with Chicken Spring Lake (and camping) shortly before reaching Cottonwood Pass. Here the PCT continues south, while you turn east (left) and descend to Horseshoe Meadows. Initially there are switchbacks, while lower you cross stretches of meadow and long sandy flats.

Maps: USGS *Mt. Whitney, Johnson Peak,* and *Cirque Lake;* TH *Mt. Whitney High Country*

Nearby Towns

The following towns are accessible from the JMT lateral trails. They are listed from north to south. Yosemite Area Regional Transit System (YARTS) buses stop in Yosemite Valley, Tuolumne Meadows, Lee Vining, June Lake, and Mammoth Lakes. Eastern Sierra Transit (EST) buses stop in Lee Vining south through Lone Pine. For the towns not described elsewhere, I've included the location of bus stops. See the map on pages 4–5 for the locations of these towns.

Yosemite Valley Lodging, restaurants, campgrounds, groceries, mountaineering and sporting goods store, and post office. See page 19 for a map and more details.

Tuolumne Meadows (Yosemite National Park) Lodging, small café, campground, groceries, small mountaineering and sporting goods store, and post office. See page 21 for a map and more details.

Lee Vining Small town with lodging, restaurants, groceries, and post office. Southbound EST buses stop at the Chevron station, and northbound EST buses stop at the Caltrans maintenance yard. YARTS buses stop at the Tioga Mobil Mart just south of town.

June Lake   Small town with lodging, restaurants, campgrounds, groceries, and post office. EST buses stop at the intersection of US 395 and CA 158. YARTS buses stop at the Rush Creek Trailhead.

Mammoth Lakes   Town with ample lodging, restaurants, campgrounds, groceries, mountaineering and sporting goods stores, and post office. Ranks with Bishop as your best choice if you must go out to a town to purchase supplies. EST buses stop at McDonald's (near the east end of Mammoth Lakes), and YARTS buses stop at many locations, including the Mammoth Mountain Inn and Shilo Inn.

Bishop   Town with ample lodging, restaurants, campgrounds, groceries, mountaineering and sporting goods stores, and post office. Ranks with Mammoth Lakes as your best choice if you must go out to a town to purchase supplies. EST buses stop at 1200 North Main Street, the Kmart parking lot.

Big Pine   Small town with lodging, restaurants, campground, some groceries, and post office. EST buses stop on Main Street, near the center of town.

Independence   Small town with lodging, restaurants, campground, some groceries, and post office. Southbound EST buses stop at the post office, and northbound EST buses stop at the courthouse.

Lone Pine   Small town with lodging, restaurants, some groceries, small mountaineering and sporting goods stores, and post office. EST buses stop at the McDonald's at 601 South Main Street. See page 22 for a map and more details.

APPENDIX B

CAMPSITES

The following table provides a selection of campsites along the JMT. It is not comprehensive, but it includes most campsites that are visible from the trail. Lacking fire rings, campsites above treeline tend to be smaller and more hidden; a few are included here, but the selection of high-elevation campsites is more sparing because many cannot sustain daily use, as would occur if they were listed here; more choices are available with a little searching. Remember that these are the coordinates where you leave the trail, not where you camp. You must be 100 feet from trail and water to camp (or 25 feet for established campsites in Kings Canyon and Sequoia National Parks). UTM coordinates indicate the location to leave the trail. If a campsite is significantly off the trail, the actual campsite location is given in parentheses. A disclaimer: UTM coordinates may be off by as much as 50 feet (15 meters), especially in deep canyons or forested areas. And remember that your GPS may also be off a little.

CAMP ID	N-S	S-N	ELEVATION	UTM COORDINATES (NAD 27)	DESCRIPTION
1.01	4.5	216.3	6,130'	11S 278399E 4179019N	large camping area in eastern Little Yosemite Valley; toilet, food-storage boxes
1.02	6.3	214.5	7,140'	11S 279291E 4180145N	many small sites to south of trail in white fir and Jeffrey pine forest
1.03	6.5	214.3	7,160'	11S 279437E 4180164N	many small sites to south of trail in white fir and Jeffrey pine forest; also small sites on the knob to the northwest of the Clouds Rest Trail junction
1.04	6.6	214.2	7,200'	11S 279547E 4180132N	large camping area by Sunrise Creek; head south from the JMT along a use trail

CAMP ID	N-S	S-N	ELEVATION	UTM COORDINATES (NAD 27)	DESCRIPTION
1.05	6.7	214.1	7,250'	11S 279655E 4180205N	site for several tents on knob with open Jeffrey pine cover and excellent views to Half Dome; head west from trail
1.06	7.1	213.7	7,430'	11S 280215E 4180266N (11S 280236E 4180229N)	large opening in Jeffrey pine/white fir forest to the south of the trail
1.07	7.2	213.6	7,470'	11S 280326E 4180338N (11S 280277E 4180367N)	head up use trail to the north; sites with excellent vistas to the west and more sheltered sites in Jeffrey pine/white fir forest to the east
1.08	8.0	212.8	7,800'	11S 281372E 4180917N	site for several tents on a little knob with Jeffrey pines above side creek; east of trail
1.09	8.1	212.7	7,830'	11S 281348E 4181052N	large opening west of creek in white fir forest; nice site
1.10	10.2	210.6	8,500'	11S 283997E 4182176N	large opening in fir forest next to a side creek; may need to detour to Sunrise Creek for water during late season
1.11	10.4	210.4	8,550'	11S 284011E 4182434N	large opening in dense fir forest alongside Sunrise Creek; head west of the trail; additional sites farther upstream to the east of the trail
1.12 Ⓧ	11.7	209.1	9,710'	11S 284852E 4183800N	large, flat, sandy site to the southeast of the trail; beautiful views but no water
1.13 Ⓧ	11.9	208.9	9,600'	11S 285079E 4184075N	site for 3–4 tents beneath open lodgepole pines at the edge of a large meadow; head south of the trail; uncertain late-season water
1.14 Ⓧ	12.1	208.7	9,580'	11S 285361E 4184157N	site for 3–4 tents beneath open lodgepole pines at the edge of a large meadow; head south of the trail; uncertain late-season water
1.15 Ⓧ	12.2	208.6	9,600'	11S 285538E 4184288N	large, flat, sandy site to the southeast of the trail; beautiful views but no water
1.16	12.8	208.0	9,320'	11S 285633E 4184995N	site for 1 tent beneath hemlocks and lodgepole pines to the northeast of the trail and creek; excellent views
1.17	13.2	207.6	9,310'	11S 285842E 4185489N (11S 285759E 4185557N)	Sunrise High Sierra Camp camping area; large area with many tent sites, a water tap, and toilet; head a short distance along the trail toward Sunrise Lakes to reach this point
1.18 Ⓧ	16.8	204.0	9,610'	11S 287693E 4190281N	openings in lodgepole pine forest and sandy flats along the southern side of Upper Cathedral Lake; do not camp in the meadow
1.19 Ⓧ	17.2	203.6	9,610'	11S 287733E 4190733N	openings in lodgepole pine forest and sandy flats along the northwest side of Upper Cathedral Lake

Ⓧ = no fires allowed

CAMP ID	N-S	S-N	ELEVATION	UTM COORDINATES (NAD 27)	DESCRIPTION
1.20 ⊗	17.7	203.1	9,430'	11S 287620E 4191522N (11S 286783E 4191387N)	many picturesque sites along the northern shore of Lower Cathedral Lake, 0.5 mile down the side trail
2.01	22.8	198.0	8,590'	11S 293123E 4194590N (11S 293077E 4194157N)	Tuolumne Meadows backpacker's campground; food-storage boxes, water, and toilets; $5 per person
2.02	28.2	192.6	8,840'	11S 298951E 4190552N	avalanche zone that marks beginning of legal camping in Lyell Canyon; hunt for options to the west of the trail, but there is no camping in the meadow
2.03	29.0	191.8	8,860'	11S 299293E 4189384N	large area under open lodgepole pine cover west of the trail
2.04	29.4	191.4	8,890'	11S 299483E 4188822N	very large area to the northwest of the Evelyn Lake junction in lodgepole pine forest
2.05	29.8	191.0	8,910'	11S 299725E 4188229N	site for 4 tents in shaded location to east of trail (toward river)
2.06	30.6	190.2	8,930'	11S 300362E 4187209N (11S 300371E 4187162N)	space for 3 tents on knob to the south of the trail
2.07	31.8	189.0	8,990'	11S 300897E 4185489N	large opening in lodgepole pine forest to the west of trail; additional smaller sites nearby; views to Mt. Lyell and Mt. Maclure from adjacent meadow
2.08	32.1	188.7	8,990'	11S 300842E 4185065N	site for 1 tent under lodgepole pine cover to the west of trail
2.09	32.4	188.4	9,070'	11S 300838E 4184616N	large area on flat shelf to the north of the trail; continue well over 100' from the trail for the best sites
2.10 ⊗	33.3	187.5	9,700'	11S 300787E 4183634N	sites for several tents on shelf above river among hemlocks and lodgepole pines; head northeast from the trail; this site is well northwest of the bridge crossing; absolutely no fires!
2.11 ⊗	33.4	187.4	9,670'	11S 300827E 4183479N	large shaded flat as one descends toward the Lyell Fork bridge; absolutely no fires!
2.12 ⊗	33.5	187.3	9,650'	11S 300871E 4183356N	2 spur trails head northeast from the southeastern side of the Lyell Fork bridge; both lead to large campsites; absolutely no fires!
2.13 ⊗	34.4	186.4	10,190'	11S 301332E 4182281N	sites for many tents beneath stunted whitebark pines to the east and northeast of the trail
2.14 ⊗	35.0	185.8	10,540'	11S 301123E 4181581N	head south from the trail to find scattered small sandy patches among slabs
3.01 ⊗	37.6	183.2	10,380'	11S 303573E 4181491N	1 well-used sandy site about 300' north of the trail; other options if you poke around; beautiful landscape of meadows and scattered whitebark pines
3.02 ⊗	38.4	182.4	10,150'	11S 304201E 4180740N	several sandy spots among slabs with scattered trees

CAMP ID		N–S	S–N	ELEVATION	UTM COORDINATES (NAD 27)	DESCRIPTION
3.03	⊗	38.7	182.1	10,070'	11S 304464E 4180314N	several sandy spots among slabs with scattered trees
3.04	⊗	38.8	182.0	10,060'	11S 304492E 4180208N	site for 4 tents under lodgepole pines a little north of the Rush Creek crossing at the Marie Lakes junction
3.05	⊗	39.7	181.1	9,680'	11S 305016E 4179603N	1 tent site in forest opening
3.06	⊗	39.9	180.9	9,630'	11S 305186E 4179516N	small site between 2 creek crossings
3.07	⊗	40.9	179.9	10,120'	11S 306395E 4179023N	single tent site under tall lodgepole pines to north of trail
4.01	⊗	41.5	179.3	10,220'	11S 306875E 4178422N	many small tent sites to either side of the trail, mostly near clusters of trees or occasionally in open z sandy flats
4.02	⊗	43.0	177.8	9,830'	11S 308733E 4177711N	head west along the use trail around Thousand Island Lake's north shore to find sandy patches among granite slabs; camping prohibited within 0.25 mile of outlet
4.03	⊗	43.2	177.6	9,820'	11S 308911E 4177556N	head west along the use trail along Thousand Island Lake's south shore; hunt for open sandy sites once past the first peninsula (camping is prohibited within 0.25 mile of the lake's outlet)
4.04	⊗	43.5	177.3	9,900'	11S 309171E 4177272N	1–2 tent sites at the edge of a small meadow southwest of the trail (above Emerald Lake)
4.05	⊗	43.8	177.0	9,940'	11S 309552E 4177027N	1 tent site on a shelf at the north end of Ruby Lake; head west from the trail
4.06	⊗	43.9	176.9	9,920'	11S 309753E 4176911N	a few small sites under hemlock trees to the southeast of Ruby Lake's outlet
4.07	⊗	45.1	175.7	9,730'	11S 310198E 4176013N	large area that can accommodate multiple parties between the trail and Garnet Lake; continue farther west around the lake for more options, looking both in forested areas and on sandy flats
4.08	⊗	45.6	175.2	9,700'	11S 310421E 4175818N	small sites along the southern shore of Garnet Lake near the island (which marks the first legal camping since the northern shore)
4.09	⊗	45.8	175.0	9,770'	11S 310343E 4175653N	sites for 2 tents in a small grove of hemlocks to the east of the trail; also sites below the trail and even more options if you descend to the lakeshore
4.10	⊗	46.3	174.5	10,110'	11S 310498E 4175326N	1 quite small site on the top of bluffs
4.11	⊗	47.9	172.9	9,190'	11S 310678E 4173859N	large open sites under a mixture of lodgepole pines, western white pines, and hemlocks to the edge of the creek (west of the trail); uncertain late-season water

⊗ = no fires allowed

CAMP ID	N–S	S–N	ELEVATION	UTM COORDINATES (NAD 27)	DESCRIPTION
4.12 🚫	48.2	172.6	9,100'	11S 310869E 4173637N	large open sites under a mixture of lodgepole pines, western white pines, and hemlocks to the edge of the creek (west of the trail); surrounded by small granite outcrops; uncertain late-season water
4.13 🚫	48.4	172.4	8,990'	11S 311102E 4173450N	a big open site on a bluff above the river; to the north of the trail just east of the Ediza Lake junction
4.14	50.5	170.3	9,400'	11S 312738E 4173192N	site for 1–2 tents close to Rosalie Lake's shore; descend to lake on a steep use trail
4.15	50.7	170.1	9,360'	11S 313032E 4173116N	several sites shaded by hemlocks to the southeast of Rosalie Lake's outlet; additional options 150' farther south along the trail (all campsites east of the trail)
4.16	51.3	169.5	9,580'	11S 313166E 4172571N	small site under lodgepole pines along Gladys Lake's north shore; head east from the trail
4.17	52.4	168.4	9,410'	11S 313718E 4171487N	large sandy sites to the west of the trail; this entire area was decimated by the 2011 windstorm
4.18	52.7	168.1	9,300'	11S 313999E 4171135N	flat knob with lodgepole pines that lies between the trail and the lake; head west from the trail
4.19	55.9	164.9	8,100'	11S 315137E 4167957N	small site in open lodgepole pine forest to the north of the Minaret Creek crossing; beautiful cobbled creek
4.20	56.8	164.0	7,680'	11S 315738E 4166946N (11S 316059E 4166825N)	head south and then east from the northern Devils Postpile junction to the Devils Postpile first-come, first-serve campground; do not expect to find a spot late in the day on weekends; $14 per campsite
4.21 (southbound)	59.2	161.6	7,640'	11S 316792E 4164496N (11S 316980E 4165434N)	head north from the Rainbow Falls junction to the Red's Meadow Resort and then onto the campground; follow the well-traveled trail just to the northeast of the resort area; $20 per campsite with campsites A, B, and C reserved for backpackers (also $20)
4.21 (northbound)	59.3	161.5	7,710'	11S 316898E 4164358N (11S 316980E 4165434N)	head north from the Reds Meadow junction to the Red's Meadow Resort and then onto the campground; follow the well-traveled trail just to the northeast of the resort area
4.22	62.0	158.8	8,650'	11S 318340E 4162258N	a few small sites along the southwestern slope of the northern Red Cone; head northeast from the Mammoth Pass junction
4.23	62.1	158.7	8,650'	11S 318360E 4162214N	several small sites in forest openings to the southwest of the Crater Creek crossing; area affected by blowdown, making location less appealing than before

🚫 = no fires allowed

CAMP ID		N–S	S–N	ELEVATION	UTM COORDINATES (NAD 27)	DESCRIPTION
5.01		65.0	155.8	9,100'	11S 320417E 4159162N	large sites that can hold many tents on the north side of Deer Creek; to the west of the trail; additional sites on the south side of Deer Creek
5.02	Ⓧ	70.1	150.7	9,980'	11S 325790E 4156238N	head downslope (south) from the trail to find small sites under lodgepole pines near the riverbank; parallel creek downstream to find several choices
5.03	Ⓧ	70.2	150.6	10,010'	11S 325837E 4156284N	2–3 small tent sites under lodgepole pines; head east toward the river; beautiful views to the Silver Divide
5.04	Ⓧ	70.3	150.5	10,020'	11S 325988E 4156299N	1 small site in trees south of the trail; site not visible from the trail
5.05	Ⓧ	72.6	148.2	9,970'	11S 327752E 4155143N	small site just near the use trail around the west side of Purple Lake; additional sites farther along the edge of Purple Lake, but fewer than previously due to 2011 blowdown
5.06	Ⓧ	74.4	146.4	10,390'	11S 328897E 4153694N	1 site for 3–4 tents and several smaller sites among whitebark pines on a long, low ridge to the north of the trail
5.07	Ⓧ	74.6	146.2	10,340'	11S 329090E 4153664N	several small sites among whitebark pines on slight knobs to the south of the trail
5.08	Ⓧ	76.9	143.9	9,510'	11S 329800E 4151887N	site for 2 small tents between the trail and Fish Creek
5.09	Ⓧ	77.0	143.8	9,490'	11S 329681E 4151743N	medium-size sloping site in open lodgepole pine forest along a stretch of Cascade Creek with big pools and slabs; north of (above) the trail
5.10	Ⓧ	77.7	143.1	9,210'	11S 329249E 4151040N	site for 3 tents in hemlock and fir forest, bit south of Fish Creek bridge; head west of the trail
5.11	Ⓧ	77.8	143.0	9,200'	11S 329201E 4150946N	site for 2 tents on open sandy knob just north of Cascade Valley (Fish Creek) junction; head west of the trail
5.12	Ⓧ	78.4	142.4	9,500'	11S 329052E 4150512N	small sites among heath vegetation and hemlocks on a small bench; west of the trail; water in gully below
5.13	Ⓧ	78.4	142.4	9,510'	11S 328997E 4150443N	2 tiny sites among heath vegetation and hemlocks on a small bench; west of the trail; water in gully below
5.14	Ⓧ	78.9	141.9	9,740'	11S 329012E 4149830N	several big sites beneath scattered lodgepole pines to edge of small marsh; south of trail
5.15	Ⓧ	79.1	141.7	9,860'	11S 329191E 4149663N	1–2 tent sites beneath scattered lodgepole pines; to south of trail
5.16	Ⓧ	80.0	140.8	10,290'	11S 329931E 4149425N	small sandy sites among slabs, mostly on the northeast side of Squaw Lake outlet; open views and evening sun

CAMP ID	N-S	S-N	ELEVATION	UTM COORDINATES (NAD 27)	DESCRIPTION
5.17 ⊗	80.6	140.2	10,540'	11S 329563E 4148911N	walk 100' from the trail (and water) and search for sandy spots that hold a single tent; the options are not visible from the trail
6.01 ⊗	82.4	138.4	10,440'	11S 330404E 4147228N	small sandy sites beneath pines scattered near the eastern shore of Silver Pass Lake; head west from trail
6.02	83.8	137.0	9,790'	11S 330076E 4145555N	several sites, each for 1–2 tents along Silver Pass Creek under scattered lodgepole pines; head west from trail
6.03	84.3	136.5	9,640'	11S 330724E 4145272N	several large sites, including a stock camp, across the large meadow; look on low knobs in the meadow for options; difficult to access during high water
6.04	85.2	135.6	8,990'	11S 331344E 4145016N	small site beneath forest cover near the Mott Lake junction; head west from trail
6.05	85.4	135.4	8,920'	11S 331289E 4144649N	2 tent sites under lodgepole pines between the trail and the creek; at the edge of Pocket Meadow
6.06	85.6	135.2	8,900'	11S 331220E 4144491N	space for several tents under lodgepole pines between the trail and the creek; at the southern end of Pocket Meadow where the creek is beginning to flow over slabs again
6.07	85.7	135.1	8,860'	11S 331150E 4144249N	site for a few tents on the west side of the creek under lodgepole pines; only accessible during low water
6.08	86.7	134.1	8,320'	11S 330975E 4143090N	site for 3–4 tents in open Jeffrey pine forest opening to the south of the trail
6.09	87.4	133.4	7,970'	11S 330604E 4142489N	site for 2 tents in white fir forest on the south side of Silver Pass Creek
6.10	87.4	133.4	7,960'	11S 330589E 4142519N	room for several tents in a shaded opening on the north side of Silver Pass Creek
6.11	88.1	132.7	7,880'	11S 329855E 4142137N	site for a few tents on an open flat with Jeffrey pines and junipers; head east of the trail
6.12	88.1	132.7	7,890'	11S 329825E 4142088N	big area on an open bench overlooking Mono Creek; to the west of the trail
6.13	93.5	127.3	9,300'	11S 331561E 4138309N	3 tent spots on a knob shaded by large Jeffrey pines and junipers to the south of the trail; uncertain late-season water
6.14	94.0	126.8	9,080'	11S 332005E 4137951N	2 small tent sites to the west of the trail
6.15	94.8	126.0	8,940'	11S 332846E 4137180N	large area on the north side of Bear Creek; follow the Bear Creek Trail west
6.16	95.0	125.8	8,990'	11S 333115E 4136988N	4 tent spots on slabs and sand between the trail and Bear Creek

CAMP ID	N–S	S–N	ELEVATION	UTM COORDINATES (NAD 27)	DESCRIPTION
6.17	95.3	125.5	9,090'	11S 333381E 4136567N	space for 3–4 tents in a lodgepole pine–covered flat between the trail and Bear Creek
6.18	95.4	125.4	9,080'	11S 333397E 4136452N	sites for at least 4 tents under lodgepole pines between the trail and Bear Creek
6.19	95.9	124.9	9,160'	11S 333630E 4135826N	site for 3–4 tents in a lodgepole pine–covered flat; head east from trail, away from Bear Creek
6.20	96.3	124.5	9,230'	11S 333765E 4135263N	large area under lodgepole pines between the trail and Bear Creek; tent sites dispersed and numerous
6.21	96.6	124.2	9,280'	11S 333762E 4134754N	2–3 tent sites in lodgepole pine forest between Bear Creek and trail
6.22	96.8	124.0	9,320'	11S 333918E 4134609N	site in open lodgepole pine forest just south of the Hilgard Branch
6.23	97.9	122.9	9,580'	11S 334689E 4133057N	spaces for 2 tents at the border of forest and expansive slabs; head west from trail
6.24	98.0	122.8	9,570'	11S 334645E 4132938N	several tent sites along the eastern bank of Bear Creek, south of the trail
6.25 🚫	99.0	121.8	10,020'	11S 334417E 4131831N	several sites, each for 2–3 tents on the low knob to the east of the trail
6.26 🚫	99.3	121.5	10,030'	11S 334188E 4131442N	open site for 2 tents to the east of the trail; also a large site a short distance along the Rose Lake Trail
6.27 🚫	100.7	120.1	10,570'	11S 334221E 4129672N	a few small sites, always for 1–2 tents, under whitebark pines around the western shore of Marie Lake; ensure you are 100' from water
7.01 🚫	102.5	118.3	10,570'	11S 333869E 4127470N	site for 1–2 tents on open slabs near Heart Lake's outlet; head west from trail
7.02 🚫	103.2	117.6	10,220'	11S 333771E 4126784N	2 tent sites on open knob east of Upper Sallie Keyes Lake; head west from trail
7.03 🚫	103.4	117.4	10,190'	11S 333812E 4126598N	large area in lodgepole pine forest between the 2 Sallie Keyes Lakes; head west from trail
7.04 🚫	103.6	117.2	10,190'	11S 333726E 4126332N	sites for many tents in lodgepole pine forest to the north of the outlet of Sallie Keyes Lakes
7.05 🚫	104.5	116.3	10,010'	11S 333867E 4125239N	large open area under scattered lodgepole pines; water in nearby meadow
7.06 🚫	104.8	116.0	10,100'	11S 334037E 4125007N	sites for 4+ tents on knob ringed by lodgepole pines with a beautiful view; water is along the trail just to the south
7.07	105.8	115.0	9,740'	11S 334706E 4124395N	small site in lodgepole pine forest along the southern bank of Senger Creek; head west from trail

🚫 = no fires allowed

CAMP ID	N-S	S-N	ELEVATION	UTM COORDINATES (NAD 27)	DESCRIPTION
7.08	107.9	111.1	7,700'	11S 334050E 4123185N or 11S 334958E 4121342N (11S 333302E 4122384N)	many sites beneath scattered trees and in sandy spots on slabs near Blayney Hot Springs; just before Muir Trail Ranch you reach a junction and head left (south) along the use trail toward the river
7.09	107.9	111.1	7,800'	11S 334050E 4123185N or 11S 334958E 4121342N (11S 334425E 4121699N)	slightly sloping bench with room for 2 tents on a shelf along the South Fork of the San Joaquin River; on southern cutoff trail to Muir Trail Ranch
7.10	107.9	111.1	7,800'	11S 334050E 4123185N or 11S 334958E 4121342N (11S 334525E 4121555N)	lodgepole pine flat with room for several tents along the South Fork of the San Joaquin River; on southern cutoff trail to Muir Trail Ranch
7.11	111.5	109.3	8,060'	11S 337471E 4121235N	site beneath open Jeffrey pines on the southeast side of the bridge at the Piute Pass junction
7.12	111.5	109.3	8,050'	11S 337507E 4121196N	large sites in sandy openings beneath junipers, Jeffrey pines, and white firs; head west from the trail
7.13	111.7	109.1	8,070'	11S 337720E 4121059N	space for 2–3 tents on lodgepole pine flat along the creek; head west from trail
7.14	111.9	108.9	8,110'	11S 337987E 4120836N	site for 3 tents on sandy shelf above the creek; head west from trail
7.15	112.9	107.9	8,230'	11S 338923E 4119903N	sandy, open spot with space for 2 tents; just west of the trail
7.16	113.0	107.8	8,250'	11S 339017E 4119840N	tiny sandy spot that holds 1 tent; just west of the trail
7.17	113.0	107.8	8,240'	11S 339105E 4119796N	room for 2 tents on a lodgepole pine–shaded shelf above the river; head west from the trail
7.18	114.1	106.7	8,390'	11S 340259E 4118713N	very large area with room for many groups in lodgepole pine forest; from the southwest side of the bridge, head north on a spur trail
7.19	114.3	106.5	8,420'	11S 340410E 4118493N	space for several tents in an open area ringed by scattered trees; just east of the trail
7.20	114.9	105.9	8,470'	11S 340709E 4117643N	big area up a small hill to the west of the trail; used as a stock camp
7.21	115.0	105.8	8,480'	11S 340786E 4117577N	space for several groups in open lodgepole pine stands along the southeastern side of the river; head south from the east side of the bridge
7.22	115.2	105.6	8,480'	11S 340783E 4117874N	large area under lodgepole pine cover just before the switchbacks to Evolution Valley begin
7.23	116.4	104.4	9,190'	11S 341729E 4117814N	small, sandy spots for 3–4 tents on a bluff above the trail; head south on a steep use trail
7.24	116.8	104.0	9,240'	11S 342109E 4117988N	small spot on bench shaded by lodgepole pines; between trail and river
7.25	116.9	103.9	9,240'	11S 342286E 4117985N	large opening ringed by lodgepole pines (stock camp); between trail and river

CAMP ID	N-S	S-N	ELEVATION	UTM COORDINATES (NAD 27)	DESCRIPTION
7.26	117.2	103.6	9,240'	11S 342682E 4117873N	sites for 3 tents in opening between the trail and Evolution Meadow
7.27	117.3	103.5	9,240'	11S 343886E 4117336N	small site beneath scattered lodgepole pines; to the north of the trail
7.28	118.1	102.7	9,470'	11S 344611E 4117057N	2–3 tent sites on sandy shelf; between trail and river
7.29	118.7	102.1	9,540'	11S 345069E 4116998N	open lodgepole pine flat at the western edge of McClure Meadow; between trail and river
7.30	119.0	101.8	9,630'	11S 345128E 4116984N	several medium-size sites at the western end of McClure Meadow, with beautiful views to Mt. Darwin and the Hermit; additional sites 100–200' farther east along trail
7.31	119.3	101.5	9,650'	11S 345497E 4116932N	several small- to large-size sites toward the eastern end of McClure Meadow, with beautiful views to Mt. Darwin and the Hermit
7.32	119.7	101.1	9,680'	11S 346123E 4116652N	2–3 tent sites in opening in lodgepole pine forest; stretch of river with pools and small cascades
7.33	120.0	100.8	9,740'	11S 346431E 4116516N	large site in a lodgepole pine flat; between the trail and river
7.34	121.4	99.4	9,940'	11S 347937E 4115348N	site for 2–3 tents on open slabs just south of the Darwin Bench drainage; views to the Hermit; between trail and river
7.35 Ⓧ	122.9	97.9	10,830'	11S 348924E 4115318N	space for 1–2 tents among whitebark pines at a tarn below Evolution Lake; head downslope (east) from the trail
7.36 Ⓧ	123.1	97.7	10,860'	11S 349130E 4115124N	sandy site for 1–2 tents among slabs to the south of the trail; make sure you use a previously used site
7.37 Ⓧ	125.1	95.7	10,980'	11S 349525E 4112936N	many options along the eastern shore of Sapphire Lake; cross the lake's outlet and walk along the eastern shore, ensuring you are 100' from water and not camped on any plants
7.38 Ⓧ	127.0	93.8	11,430'	11S 349306E 4110304N	space for ~5 small tents, distributed over a large area near the Wanda Lake outlet; each site is small, sandy, and surrounded by slabs; beautiful views
7.39 Ⓧ	127.7	93.1	11,460'	11S 350097E 4109536N	space for 2 tents on the shallow ridge that separates the trail from Wanda Lake; lovely views of Evolution Basin
8.01 Ⓧ	129.6	91.2	11,690'	11S 352132E 4108629N (11S 352105E 4108700N)	sandy site for 1–2 tents among slabs next to a small tarn above Helen Lake; head 200' northwest from the trail
8.02 Ⓧ	131.2	89.6	11,150'	11S 353543E 4109680N	space for 1 tent in a sandy patch on a whitebark pine–covered knob
8.03 Ⓧ	132.0	88.8	10,840'	11S 354190E 4109551N	2 sandy tent sites at the southeastern edge of Lake 10,800+; excellent views

Ⓧ = no fires allowed

CAMP ID	N-S	S-N	ELEVATION	UTM COORDINATES (NAD 27)	DESCRIPTION
8.04 ⊗	132.0	88.8	10,850'	11S 354255E 4109426N	big site on shelf to the east of the creek
8.05 ⊗	132.3	88.5	10,700'	11S 354266E 4109185N	2 tent sites in small opening beneath whitebark pines; head east from the trail
8.06 ⊗	132.4	88.4	10,640'	11S 354389E 4109048N	1 tent site under lodgepole pines to the west of the trail; good views to the Black Giant
8.07 ⊗	132.7	88.1	10,470'	11S 354408E 4108809N	lodgepole pine flat above river with space for quite a few tents; good views to the Black Giant; head west from trail
8.08 ⊗	133.0	87.8	10,320'	11S 354628E 4108612N	Starrs Camp; at least 5 tent sites among young lodgepole pines to the south of the trail; beautiful views of Langille Peak, the Black Giant, and Le Conte Canyon
8.09	134.2	86.6	9,480'	11S 356026E 4108399N	sites for 5 tents beside creek just south of the switchbacks
8.10	134.5	86.3	9,380'	11S 356447E 4108399N	2–3 tent sites on sandy bench above river
8.11	134.8	86.0	9,310'	11S 356939E 4108489N	large area under lodgepole pine cover between the trail and river
8.12	135.2	85.6	9,250'	11S 357367E 4108394N	space for many tents (across several small sites) in openings in lodgepole pine forest; just south of Big Pete Creek crossing
8.13	135.4	85.4	9,230'	11S 357585E 4108192N	Big Pete Meadow; lateral trail to large site by creek under lodgepole pine cover
8.14	135.8	85.0	9,010'	11S 357827E 4107654N	space for 1–2 tents on a sandy shelf with excellent views of Langille Peak and to the south; head west from trail
8.15	136.1	84.7	8,860'	11S 357968E 4107320N	site for 2 tents under lodgepole pines; head west from trail
8.16	136.2	84.6	8,860'	11S 358043E 4107208N	Little Pete Meadow; big stock camp under lodgepole pine cover at edge of meadow; head west from trail
8.17	136.9	83.9	8,740'	11S 358394E 4106307N (11S 358437E 4106267N)	2 sites in sandy flats among slabs with good views; walk a short distance up the Bishop Pass Trail (to coordinates) and then head south
8.18	136.9	83.9	8,720'	11S 358405E 4106254N	big areas under lodgepole pines; head west from trail
8.19	137.0	83.8	8,710'	11S 358413E 4106202N	space for 5 tents under lodgepole pines; head west from trail; additional site closer to the Dusy Fork bridge
8.20	137.1	83.7	8,690'	11S 358390E 4105977N	spot for 1–2 tents under lodgepole pines; head east from trail
8.21	137.3	83.5	8,640'	11S 358282E 4105738N	spot for 1–2 tents under lodgepole pines; head west from trail
8.22	137.4	83.4	8,640'	11S 358319E 4105633N	site for 2–3 tents under lodgepole pines with views to the Citadel; head west from trail
8.23	138.3	82.5	8,350'	11S 358159E 4104265N	space for 3 tents on open bench above river; head west from trail

CAMP ID	N-S	S-N	ELEVATION	UTM COORDINATES (NAD 27)	DESCRIPTION
8.24	139.3	81.5	8,240'	11S 358792E 4102912N	space for 5 tents at the edge of Grouse Meadow; head west from trail
8.25	139.3	81.5	8,250'	11S 358854E 4102835N	space for 3 tents at the edge of Grouse Meadow; head west from trail
8.26	139.4	81.4	8,240'	11S 358908E 4102796N	site for 1 tent under lodgepole pines near the edge of Grouse Meadow; head east from trail
8.27	140.3	80.5	8,050'	11S 359614E 4101718N	several large sites beneath Jeffrey pines at the Middle Fork Trail junction; head south from trail
8.28	141.4	79.4	8,430'	11S 361063E 4101688N	2 tent sites on shelf above creek with some lodgepole pine cover; head south from trail
8.29	141.6	79.2	8,430'	11S 361299E 4101671N	2 small tent sites under Jeffrey pines; head north from trail
8.30	143.0	77.8	8,680'	11S 363369E 4101721N	site for 4+ tents on lodgepole pine flat between trail and river; pocket of trees within the burn area
8.31	143.3	77.5	8,730'	11S 363705E 4101859N	space for 4 tents in lodgepole pine flat between trail and river; pocket of trees within the burn area
8.32	143.8	77.0	8,870'	11S 364434E 4101985N	Deer Meadow; very large site beneath lodgepole pine forest just east of creek crossing draining Palisade Basin; head south from trail
8.33	144.3	76.5	8,890'	11S 365009E 4101799N	large areas under lodgepole pines and big red firs near the base of the Golden Staircase; head south from trail
8.34	144.4	76.4	8,960'	11S 365252E 4101832N	2–3 tent sites under lodgepole pines and red firs near the base of the Golden Staircase; head south from trail
8.35 ⊗	146.5	74.3	10,360'	11S 367067E 4101836N	space for 1–2 tents on sandy flat next to hemlocks; head southeast from trail; good views to west
8.36 ⊗	147.2	73.6	10,590'	11S 367592E 4102422N	2 tent spots in sandy patches between slabs; head south from trail
8.37 ⊗	147.3	73.5	10,600'	11S 367773E 4102386N	Lower Palisade Lake; lots of small sandy spots among slabs, both north of lake and southwest of lake at outlet; views to the Middle Palisade group
8.38 ⊗	148.2	72.6	10,790'	11S 368796E 4101960N	2 sandy sites under whitebark pines; head south from trail; additional options southeast along the trail
8.39 ⊗	148.4	72.4	10,840'	11S 369099E 4101740N	many sites near each other; all sandy spots among slabs, surrounded by whitebark pines and overlooking Upper Palisade Lake; excellent views; water a short distance south on trail

⊗ = no fires allowed

CAMP ID		N-S	S-N	ELEVATION	UTM COORDINATES (NAD 27)	DESCRIPTION
8.40	🚫	148.5	72.3	10,840'	11S 369143E 4101671N	several sandy sites with whitebark pines on the northwest side of the creek
8.41	🚫	148.6	72.2	10,850'	11S 369251E 4101490N	space for 3 tents beneath stunted whitebark pines and overlooking Upper Palisade Lake; excellent views; head west of trail
8.42	🚫	149.1	71.7	10,970'	11S 369524E 4100850N	1–2 small tent sites under last whitebark pines; amazing views down to the Palisade Lakes
9.01	🚫	152.1	68.7	11,610'	11S 370721E 4098884N	Upper Basin; head due east to reach large lake with many flat, sandy tent sites; beautiful surroundings
9.02	🚫	152.5	68.3	11,500'	11S 370468E 4098259N	wander in any direction to find sandy tent sites near the many tarns in Upper Basin; make sure you camp on unvegetated areas 100' from water
9.03		155.3	65.5	10,570'	11S 371168E 4094326N	search around for options toward stream; east of the trail
9.04	🚫	156.3	64.5	10,190'	11S 371685E 4092851N	site for 5 tents in open flat just east of trail
9.05	🚫	156.3	64.5	10,170'	11S 371672E 4092792N	from cairn marking abandoned Taboose Pass Trail, head east to creek; here there is a large opening under lodgepole pines
9.06	🚫	156.7	64.1	10,050'	11S 371502E 4092346N	several sites for 1–2 tents in lodgepole pine forest on the south side of the river crossing; head east from trail
9.07	🚫	156.7	64.1	10,050'	11S 371517E 4092288N	several tent sites in sandy openings to the west of the trail; farther from water than previous camp
9.08	🚫	158.1	62.7	10,860'	11S 372161E 4091060N	2–3 small tent sites just next to trail; some to the east and others to the west
9.09	🚫	158.4	62.4	11,000'	11S 372292E 4090590N	tent sites on small knob with whitebark pines; head west toward a tarn
9.10	🚫	158.7	62.1	11,050'	11S 372478E 4090187N	5+ individual tent sites in sandy spots among slabs and whitebark pines between two small lakes
9.11	🚫	158.9	61.9	11,080'	11S 372495E 4090007N	sandy site for 1 tent near the lake; head west of trail
9.12	🚫	159.1	61.7	11,130'	11S 372595E 4089730N	1–2 tent sites in sandy location near the north shore of Lake Marjorie
9.13	🚫	159.2	61.6	11,150'	11S 372766E 4089702N	a few sandy spots on either side of the trail; landscape of slabs and whitebark pines
9.14	🚫	159.5	61.3	11,250'	11S 373005E 4089464N	2 small sites among whitebark pines; head east from trail; water a short walk up the trail
9.15	🚫	159.7	61.1	11,280'	11S 373120E 4089338N	1–2 sandy spots on slab west of the trail; water a short walk down the trail
9.16	🚫	160.2	60.6	11,580'	11S 373640E 4088926N	big sandy flat below the trail; good late-season site but could be damp earlier; beautiful views

CAMP ID	N-S	S-N	ELEVATION	UTM COORDINATES (NAD 27)	DESCRIPTION
10.01 🚫	162.6	58.2	11,380'	11S 375436E 4087425N	head 500' north to the chain of small lakes; hunt for sandy flats among whitebark pines, ensuring you are camped off vegetation
10.02 🚫	163.7	57.1	10,890'	11S 375735E 4086049N	big site in an opening on a knob, surrounded by lodgepole pines; head south from the trail (away from the lake)
10.03 🚫	164.2	56.6	10,610'	11S 375520E 4085427N (11S 375607E 4085397N)	head 300' east toward the outlet of Twin Lakes; space for 2 tents beneath lodgepole pines
10.04 🚫	164.7	56.1	10,350'	11S 375315E 4084786N	small site east of Sawmill Trail junction under lodgepole pine cover with wet streamside vegetation; cross to east side of creek
10.05	165.5	55.3	9,800'	11S 374383E 4084432N	big site on a shelf shaded by lodgepole pines; head east from trail
10.06	166.6	54.2	9,240'	11S 373453E 4083300N	several tent sites on bench above river partially shaded by lodgepole pines; head south from trail
10.07	168.4	52.4	8,520'	11S 371951E 4081594N	large site just south of Woods Creek crossing with room for 20 parties; additional sites on the knob to the southwest of the trail; food-storage boxes
10.08	170.8	50.0	9,450'	11S 374029E 4079218N	several small sites under lodgepole pine cover to the east of a marshy area; head south from trail
10.09 🚫	172.4	48.4	10,220'	11S 374516E 4077255N	many sites along the north shore of Dollar Lake; beautiful reflections of Fin Dome in the lake
10.10 🚫	172.4	48.4	10,220'	11S 374487E 4077241N	sites along the west shore of Dollar Lake; head east from trail, taking note of the restoration areas
10.11 🚫	173.0	47.8	10,310'	11S 374369E 4076481N	Arrowhead Lake; first tent sites are beneath lodgepole pines near where you leave the trail; continue south, paralleling the lakeshore for many more options both under forest cover and on shady knobs even farther south; fantastic view of Fin Dome; food-storage box
10.12 🚫	173.9	46.9	10,560'	11S 374721E 4075127N	large sites in sandy flats with sparse lodgepole pine cover; on bench overlooking Lower Rae Lake
10.13 🚫	174.0	46.8	10,570'	11S 374760E 4075057N	Lower Rae Lake; large sites in sandy flats with sparse lodgepole pine cover; on bench overlooking Lower Rae Lake; food-storage box
10.14 🚫	174.2	46.6	10,590'	11S 375019E 4074783N	few small sandy sites on a shelf overlooking Middle Rae Lake
10.15 🚫	174.4	46.4	10,590'	11S 375188E 4074573N	1 tent site on sandy bench above Middle Rae Lake; beautiful views to the Painted Lady

🚫 = no fires allowed

CAMP ID	N–S	S–N	ELEVATION	UTM COORDINATES (NAD 27)	DESCRIPTION
10.16 ⊛	174.8	46.0	10,610'	11S 375377E 4074106N	Middle Rae Lake; very large camping area along the shore of Middle Rae Lake; head 500' west on a spur trail toward lake; food-storage boxes
10.17 ⊛	175.4	45.4	10,560'	11S 374963E 4073711N	~5 small sandy spots, each for 1 tent, among slabs and whitebark pines scattered around the Sixty Lake Basin junction; most sites are not visible from the trail; fantastic views of the Painted Lady and Upper Rae Lake
10.18 ⊛	176.2	44.6	11,090'	11S 374583E 4073136N	space for 2–3 tents in a cluster of whitebark pines on a knob with a tarn behind; head northwest from trail
10.19 ⊛	176.5	44.3	11,380'	11S 374331E 4072689N	exposed alpine sites in sandy patches between slabs by tarns to west of trail; sites best seen when you are slightly above them
11.01 ⊛	177.7	43.1	11,570'	11S 373961E 4071908N	several small sites among whitebark pines near the lake outlet; head east from trail
11.02 ⊛	179.6	41.2	10,740'	11S 373685E 4070166N (11S 372780E 4070952N)	large area in lodgepole pine forest at the north end of Charlotte Lake; food-storage box; 0.9 mile off the JMT on the trail to Charlotte Lake
11.03 ⊛	180.0	40.8	10,520'	11S 374110E 4069887N	small sites among streamside vegetation and foxtail pines at Bullfrog Lake Junction; head east from trail
11.04 ⊛	180.2	40.6	10,360'	11S 374160E 4069650N	site for a few tents on shelf above creek with lodgepole pine cover and wet heath vegetation; head south from trail
11.05 ⊛	180.6	40.2	10,070'	11S 374409E 4069459N	2–3 shaded tent sites under lodgepole pines to the west of the creek crossing; head south from trail
11.06	181.1	39.7	9,550'	11S 374054E 4069011N	large sites in wet (and often buggy) lodgepole pine forest just upstream of Bubbs Creek junction; head south from trail
11.07	181.4	39.4	9,530'	11S 374419E 4068919N	2 spots next to trail in dry lodgepole pine forest; just north of Vidette Meadow
11.08	181.5	39.3	9,540'	11S 374566E 4068865N	Vidette Meadow; several large sites in opening in dry lodgepole pine forest at edge of Vidette Meadow; views to East Vidette; food-storage box
11.09	181.6	39.2	9,550'	11S 374670E 4068796N	large site in dry lodgepole pine forest at edge of Vidette Meadow; views to East Vidette; more options 200' south
11.10	182.4	38.4	9,910'	11S 375616E 4068174N	Upper Vidette Meadow; large opening in flat lodgepole pine forest; food-storage box
11.11 ⊛	182.6	38.2	9,960'	11S 375833E 4068121N	large site in dry lodgepole pine forest; head west from trail
11.12 ⊛	184.0	36.8	10,400'	11S 376951E 4066475N	space for a few tents on a shelf between the trail and stream; under lodgepole pine cover

CAMP ID	N-S	S-N	ELEVATION	UTM COORDINATES (NAD 27)	DESCRIPTION
11.13 Ⓧ	184.3	36.5	10,460'	11S 377220E 4066135N	2 small sites under lodgepole pines; head east from trail
11.14 Ⓧ	184.3	36.5	10,480'	11S 377256E 4066060N	Center Basin junction; lots of sandy sites among slabs above the river and on a lodgepole pine flat; head west from trail; food-storage box
11.15 Ⓧ	184.7	36.1	10,530'	11S 377492E 4065690N	sites for ~5 tents just to the south of the Center Basin creek crossing; look to both sides of the trail
11.16 Ⓧ	185.6	35.2	10,910'	11S 377616E 4064562N	3–4 small tent sites on small knob with whitebark pines; seasonal trickle nearby; spectacular views; uncertain late-season water
11.17 Ⓧ	185.6	35.2	10,930'	11S 377584E 4064455N	3–4 small tent sites on flat shelf with scattered whitebark pines above valley; seasonal trickle nearby; spectacular views; uncertain late-season water
11.18 Ⓧ	186.1	34.7	11,230'	11S 377550E 4063727N	several single tent sites beneath last stand of foxtail pines; excellent views
11.19 Ⓧ	186.2	34.6	11,240'	11S 377587E 4063736N	a few small spots in sandy flats, mostly without tree cover; amazing views
11.20 Ⓧ	187.2	33.6	11,770'	11S 378141E 4063449N	2 small sandy tent sites among slabs and boulders near the small tarn to the east of the trail; be sure to keep off alpine plants
11.21 Ⓧ	188.1	32.7	12,240'	11S 377824E 4062542N	a few exposed tent sites overlooking Lake 12,250 and surrounded by talus; excellent views to Junction Peak
12.01 Ⓧ	190.2	30.6	12,500'	11S 377308E 4061263N	a few sandy flats among slabs near the outlet of the first lake south of Forester Pass
12.02 Ⓧ	191.1	29.7	12,270'	11S 376837E 4060044N	2 tent sites in sandy flat; open landscape; seasonal water nearby but lakes farther away
12.03 Ⓧ	191.2	29.6	12,220'	11S 376811E 4059934N	sandy tent site just southeast of the trail, with additional options if you continue to nearby lakes
12.04 Ⓧ	193.2	27.6	11,360'	11S 375960E 4057330N	1 site in big grove of foxtail pines east of the trail; seeps with water nearby but uncertain late-season water
12.05 Ⓧ	194.1	26.7	10,980'	11S 376041E 4055999N	site for 1–2 tents in sandy opening to the north of the trail
12.06 Ⓧ	194.1	26.7	10,970'	11S 376052E 4055967N	Tyndall Creek crossing; space for 4+ tents in the large sandy opening to the west of trail; search farther west and south for other options; food-storage box
12.07 Ⓧ	194.4	26.4	10,880'	11S 375984E 4055650N	several sandy sites just north of the Tyndall ranger cabin junction; head west from trail
12.08 Ⓧ	194.8	26.0	11,030'	11S 376211E 4055104N	Tyndall Frog Ponds; large sites under open lodgepole pines; look on both sides of the trail; food-storage box

Ⓧ = no fires allowed

CAMP ID	N–S	S–N	ELEVATION	UTM COORDINATES (NAD 27)	DESCRIPTION
12.09	196.0	24.8	11,430'	11S 376685E 4053326N	lots of flat, sandy spots along the northern side of the lake on Bighorn Plateau; no trees or large rocks for shelter; make sure you camp off vegetation and 100' away from the lake
12.10	197.6	23.2	10,800'	11S 377308E 4051328N	lodgepole pine–shaded sites on shelf above Wright Creek; head south from trail
12.11	197.9	22.9	10,690'	11S 377081E 4050929N	a few sites in a lodgepole pine–shaded opening to the south of Wright Creek; head west from trail; additional options another 100' to the south
12.12	198.6	22.2	10,410'	11S 377432E 4050541N	large site near the High Sierra Trail junction, adjacent to open meadow
12.13	198.7	22.1	10,400'	11S 377464E 4050477N	Wallace Creek crossing; many sites under scattered lodgepole pines on the southwest side of Wallace Creek; continue another 100' to the south for additional choices; food-storage box
12.14	198.8	22.0	10,460'	11S 377680E 4050493N	open sandy campsite, but it is a 500' walk to Wallace Creek for water
12.15	199.2	21.6	10,650'	11S 377495E 4050180N	2 tent sites under lodgepole pines just north of a small creek; head east from trail
12.16	200.8	20.0	10,700'	11S 377402E 4048191N	2 tent sites at edge of Sandy Meadow in mixed foxtail and lodgepole pine forest to the west of the creek crossing; head south from trail; uncertain late-season water
12.17	202.8	18.0	10,670'	11S 379142E 4047130N	large site under lodgepole pine forest to the east of trail
12.18	202.9	17.9	10,770'	11S 379241E 4047243N	Crabtree camping area; head south along the spur trail, across the creek to a large number of sites ringing the meadow; food-storage box and toilet
12.19	203.5	17.3	11,110'	11S 379954E 4047528N	small tent sites on open sandy bench above creek; head south from trail
12.20	204.7	16.1	11,570'	11S 381322E 4047603N	3 tent spots under lodgepole pines between trail and creek
12.21	205.7	15.1	11,490'	11S 382326E 4048136N	head south to find sandy sites on the knob north of Guitar Lake and toward the west end of the lake; beautiful views to the Kaweahs and Mt. Whitney
12.22	205.8	15.0	11,500'	11S 382505E 4048032N	many exposed, sandy sites among slabs near the north shore of Guitar Lake; alpine scenery and beautiful views to Mt. Whitney; head southwest from the trail
12.23	206.5	14.3	11,910'	11S 382629E 4047999N	few small tent sites in sandy flats among slabs above Guitar Lake; head south from trail once east of Arctic Creek
12.24	206.6	14.2	11,920'	11S 383443E 4047422N	walk a short distance south to find sandy flats between many small tarns; uncertain late-season water

CAMP ID	N–S	S–N	ELEVATION	UTM COORDINATES (NAD 27)	DESCRIPTION
12.25 🚫	208.2	12.6	13,280'	11S 384291E 4046766N	space for 1 tent on an exposed patch of sand with steep bluffs below; no water
12.26 🚫	208.3	12.5	13,400'	11S 384334E 4046822N	room for 5 small tents in sandy spots among talus, mostly sheltered by rock walls; amazing views to the west; head east (upslope) from the trail on the last switchback below the Mt. Whitney trail junction; no water
12.27 🚫	210.4	10.4	14,505'	11S 384473E 4048700N	Mt. Whitney summit; various sandy flats among boulders; views in all directions!; no water
13.01 🚫	214.7	6.1	12,040'	11S 385616E 4046956N	Trail Camp; many sites in sandy flats among slabs, on both sides of trail
13.02 🚫	214.8	6.0	11,990'	11S 385773E 4047005N	a few sandy sites among slabs at the far eastern end of Trail Camp
13.03 🚫	215.6	5.2	11,430'	11S 386654E 4047420N	1–2 small sandy tent sites among slabs on open knob
13.04 🚫	216.2	4.6	10,900'	11S 387116E 4047520N	small open sites on knob; excellent views but far from water
13.05 🚫	216.3	4.5	10,840'	11S 387140E 4047638N	medium-size site beneath sparse tree cover; excellent views but far from water
13.06 🚫	217.0	3.8	10,370'	11S 387445E 4047888N	Outpost Camp; very large area beneath scattered foxtail pines
13.07 🚫	217.9	2.9	10,010'	11S 388197E 4048255N	little-used camping choices near the shores of Lone Pine Lake; head east along the spur trail for 0.2 mile to reach the lake

🚫 = no fires allowed
North-to-south distances are in miles from Happy Isles, while south-to-north distances are in miles from Whitney Portal.

APPENDIX C

FOOD-STORAGE BOXES (BEAR BOXES)

LOCATION	ELEVATION	UTM COORDINATES (NAD27)
Little Yosemite Valley (Camp 1.01)	6,130'	11S 278409E 4179015N
Sunrise High Sierra Camp (Camp 1.17)	9,310'	11S 285790E 4185522N
south side of Woods Creek crossing (Camp 10.07)	8,530'	11S 371951E 4081607N
Arrowhead Lake (Camp 10.11)	10,300'	11S 374375E 4076443N
Lower Rae Lake (Camp 10.13)	10,560'	11S 374742E 4075037N
Middle Rae Lake (Camp 10.16)	10,560'	11S 375248E 4074161N
Charlotte Lake (Camp 11.02)	10,400'	11S 372816E 4070866N
Vidette Meadow (Camp 11.08)	9,550'	11S 374566E 4068867N
Upper Vidette Meadow (Camp 11.10)	9,945'	11S 375616E 4068176N
Center Basin junction (Camp 11.14)	10,500'	11S 377247E 4066060N
Tyndall Creek crossing (Camp 12.06)	10,965'	11S 376032E 4055967N
Tyndall Frog Ponds (Camp 12.08)	11,025'	11S 376215E 4055105N
Wallace Creek crossing (Camp 12.13)	10,400'	11S 377457E 4050483N
Crabtree Meadow (Camp 12.18)	10,700'	11S 379333E 4047146N

* The Charlotte Lake food-storage box and campsite are 0.8 mile off the JMT toward the northern end of Charlotte Lake.
**The food-storage boxes at Kearsarge Lakes have been locked; they were being abused as food-storage depots by JMT and PCT hikers.

Locations of food-storage boxes not on the JMT are available at **climber.org/data/bearboxes.html**.

APPENDIX D

PLANTS REFERENCED IN TEXT

Below and on the following pages is a table of plant names referenced in the text, indexed by scientific name (alphabetized by family).

COMMON NAME	SCIENTIFIC NAME	FAMILY
red elderberry	*Sambucus racemosa* var. *racemosa*	Adoxaceae (Caprifoliaceae)
swamp onion, Pacific mountain onion	*Allium validum*	Alliaceae (Liliaceae)
Sierra angelica	*Angelica lineariloba*	Apiaceae
wide-leaved Parish's yampah	*Perideridia parishii* ssp. *latifolia*	Apiaceae
ranger's buttons	*Sphenosciadium capitellatum*	Apiaceae
bitter dogbane	*Apocynum androsaemifolium*	Apocynaceae
western eupatorium	*Ageratina occidentalis*	Asteraceae
mountain agoseris	*Agoseris monticola*	Asteraceae
meadow pussytoes	*Antennaria corymbosa*	Asteraceae
rosy pussytoes	*Antennaria rosea* ssp. *confinis*	Asteraceae
Sierra arnica	*Arnica nevadensis*	Asteraceae
mountain big sagebrush	*Artemisia tridentata* ssp. *vaseyana*	Asteraceae
rose thistle	*Cirsium andersonii*	Asteraceae
dinnerplate thistle	*Cirsium scariosum* var. *americanum*	Asteraceae

COMMON NAME	SCIENTIFIC NAME	FAMILY
Sierra fleabane daisy	*Erigeron algidus*	Asteraceae
cutleaf fleabane daisy	*Erigeron compositus*	Asteraceae
Coulter's fleabane daisy	*Erigeron coulteri*	Asteraceae
Bigelow's sneezeweed	*Helenium bigelovii*	Asteraceae
shaggy hawkweed	*Hieracium horridum*	Asteraceae
alpine gold	*Hulsea algida*	Asteraceae
orange sneezeweed	*Hymenoxys hoopesii*	Asteraceae
tundra aster	*Oreostemma alpigenum* var. *andersonii*	Asteraceae
alpineflames	*Pyrrocoma apargioides*	Asteraceae
western dwarf mountain ragwort	*Senecio fremontii* var. *occidentalis*	Asteraceae
arrowleaf ragwort	*Senecio triangularis*	Asteraceae
alpine goldenrod	*Solidago multiradiata*	Asteraceae
rockcress	*Boechera* sp.	Brassicaceae
granite draba	*Draba lemmonii*	Brassicaceae
sanddune wallflower	*Erysimum perenne*	Brassicaceae
Nuttall's sandwort	*Minuartia nuttallii* var. *gracilis*	Caryophyllaceae
ledge stonecrop, western roseroot	*Rhodiola integrifolia* ssp. *integrifolia*	Crassulaceae
Sierra stonecrop	*Sedum obtusatum* ssp. *obtusatum*	Crassulaceae
incense cedar	*Calocedrus decurrens*	Cupressaceae
western juniper	*Juniperus occidentalis*	Cupressaceae
sedge	*Carex* sp.	Cyperaceae
Heller's sedge	*Carex helleri*	Cyperaceae
pinemat manzanita	*Arctostaphylos nevadensis* ssp. *nevadensis*	Ericaceae
greenleaf mananita	*Arctostaphylos patula*	Ericaceae
white mountain heather	*Cassiope mertensiana*	Ericaceae
mountain laurel	*Kalmia polifolia*	Ericaceae
red mountain heather	*Phyllodoce breweri*	Ericaceae
white-veined wintergreen	*Pyrola picta*	Ericaceae
western Labrador tea	*Rhododendron columbianum*	Ericaceae

COMMON NAME	SCIENTIFIC NAME	FAMILY
snowplant	*Sarcodes sanguinea*	Ericaceae
dwarf bilberry	*Vaccinium caespitosum*	Ericaceae
western blueberry	*Vaccinium uliginosum* ssp. *occidentale*	Ericaceae
matted Brewer's lupine	*Lupinus breweri* ssp. *bryoides*	Fabaceae
carpet clover	*Trifolium monanthum* ssp. *monanthum*	Fabaceae
bush chinquapin	*Chrysolepis sempervirens*	Fagaceae
huckleberry oak	*Quercus vacciniifolia*	Fagaceae
Fremont silktassel	*Garrya fremontii*	Garryaceae
alpine gentian	*Gentiana newberryi* var. *tiogana*	Gentianaceae
Sierra gentian	*Gentianopsis holopetala*	Gentianaceae
felwort	*Swertia perennis*	Gentianaceae
wax currant	*Ribes cereum* var. *inebrians*	Grossulariaceae
alpine prickly currant	*Ribes montigenum*	Grossulariaceae
Sierra gooseberry	*Ribes roezlii* var. *roezlii*	Grossulariaceae
rosy-petaled cliffbush	*Jamesia americana* var. *rosea*	Hydrangeaceae
pennyroyal, coyote mint	*Monardella odoratissima* ssp. *pallida*	Lamiaceae
California bay laurel	*Umbellularia californica*	Lauraceae
Leichtlin's mariposa lily	*Calochortus leichtlinii*	Liliaceae
Kelley's tiger lily	*Lilium kelleyanum*	Liliaceae
western blue flax	*Linum lewisii* var. *lewisii*	Linaceae
California corn lily	*Veratrum californicum* var. *californicum*	Melanthiaceae (Liliaceae)
pussypaws	*Calyptridium umbellatum*	Montiaceae (Portulacaceae)
fireweed	*Chamerion angustifolium* ssp. *circumvagum*	Onagraceae
California fuchsia	*Epilobium canum* ssp. *latifolium*	Onagraceae
rockfringe	*Epilobium obcordatum*	Onagraceae
western rattlesnake plantain	*Goodyera oblongifolia*	Orchidaceae
Sierra bog orchid	*Platanthera dilatata* var. *leucostachys*	Orchidaceae

COMMON NAME	SCIENTIFIC NAME	FAMILY
wavyleaf paintbrush	*Castilleja applegatei* ssp. *pallida*	Orobanchaceae (Scrophulariacae)
Lemmon's paintbrush	*Castilleja lemmonii*	Orobanchaceae (Scrophulariacae)
great red paintbrush	*Castilleja miniata* ssp. *miniata*	Orobanchaceae (Scrophulariacae)
dwarf alpine paintbrush, alpine paintbrush	*Castilleja nana*	Orobanchaceae (Scrophulariacae)
Peirson's paintbrush	*Castilleja peirsonii*	Orobanchaceae (Scrophulariacae)
little elephant's head	*Pedicularis attollens*	Orobanchaceae (Scrophulariacae)
marsh grass of Parnassus	*Parnassia palustris*	Parnassiaceae (Saxifragaceae)
primrose monkeyflower	*Mimulus primuloides* var. *primuloides*	Phrymaceae (Scrophulariacae)
larger mountain monkeyflower	*Mimulus tilingii*	Phrymaceae (Scrophulariacae)
white fir	*Abies concolor*	Pinaceae
red fir	*Abies magnifica*	Pinaceae
whitebark pine	*Pinus albicaulis*	Pinaceae
foxtail pine	*Pinus balfouriana*	Pinaceae
lodgepole pine	*Pinus contorta*	Pinaceae
Jeffrey pine	*Pinus jeffreyi*	Pinaceae
sugar pine	*Pinus lambertiana*	Pinaceae
singleleaf pinyon	*Pinus monophylla*	Pinaceae
western white pine	*Pinus monticola*	Pinaceae
Douglas-fir	*Pseudotsuga menziesii*	Pinaceae
mountain hemlock	*Tsuga mertensiana*	Pinaceae
azure penstemon	*Penstemon azureus*	Plataginaceae (Scrophulariacae)
Sierra penstemon	*Penstemon heterodoxus* var. *cephalophorus*	Plataginaceae (Scrophulariacae)
mountain pride penstemon	*Penstemon newberryi* var. *newberryi*	Plataginaceae (Scrophulariacae)
Bridge penstemon, scarlet penstemon	*Penstemon rostriflorus*	Plataginaceae (Scrophulariacae)
mountain meadow penstemon	*Penstemon rydbergii*	Plataginaceae (Scrophulariacae)
granite gilia	*Linanthus pungens*	Polemoniaceae

COMMON NAME	SCIENTIFIC NAME	FAMILY
spreading phlox	*Phlox diffusa*	Polemoniaceae
skypilot	*Polemonium eximium*	Polemoniaceae
western bistort	*Bistorta bistortoides*	Polygonaceae
frosted wild buckwheat	*Eriogonum incanum*	Polygonaceae
Sierra cushion wild buckwheat	*Eriogonum ovalifolium* var. *nivale*	Polygonaceae
Coville's sulphur flower	*Eriogonum umbellatum* var. *covillei*	Polygonaceae
alpine mountain sorrel	*Oxyria digyna*	Polygonaceae
mountaineer shooting star	*Dodecatheon redolens*	Primulaceae
Sierra primrose	*Primula suffrutescens*	Primulaceae
crimson columbine	*Aquilegia formosa*	Ranunculaceae
Eschscholtz's buttercup	*Ranunculus eschscholtzii* var. *oxynotus*	Ranunculaceae
mountain whitethorn	*Ceanothus cordulatus*	Rhamnaceae
curl-leaf mountain mahogany	*Cercocarpus ledifolius* var. *ledifolius*	Rosaceae
fern bush	*Chamaebatiaria millefolium*	Rosaceae
shrubby cinquefoil	*Dasiphora fruticosa*	Rosaceae
ocean spray	*Holodiscus discolor* var. *microphyllus*	Rosaceae
clubmoss ivesia	*Ivesia lycopodioides* var. *lycopodioides*	Rosaceae
Muir's ivesia	*Ivesia muirii*	Rosaceae
dwarf ivesia	*Ivesia pygmaea*	Rosaceae
Sierra mousetail	*Ivesia santolinoides*	Rosaceae
rock spiraea	*Spiraea splendens*	Rosaceae
quaking aspen	*Populus tremuloides*	Salicaceae
Rocky Mountain willow	*Salix petrophila*	Salicaceae
bigleaf maple	*Acer macrophyllum*	Sapindaceae (Aceraceae)
pink alumroot	*Heuchera rubescens*	Saxifragaceae
bud saxifrage	*Micranthes bryophora*	Saxifragaceae
brook saxifrage	*Micranthes odontoloma*	Saxifragaceae
Tolmie's saxifrage	*Micranthes tolmiei*	Saxifragaceae
mountain prettyface	*Triteleia ixioides* ssp. *anilina*	Themidaceae (Liliaceae)

APPENDIX E

BIBLIOGRAPHY AND
SUGGESTED READING

Arnold, Daniel. *Early Days in the Range of Light: Encounters with Legendary Mountaineers.* Berkeley, CA: Counterpoint Press, 2009.

Beedy, Edward C., and Edward R. Pandolfino. *Birds of the Sierra Nevada: Their Natural History, Status, and Distribution.* Berkeley, CA: University of California Press, 2013.

Beffort, Brian. *Joy of Backpacking.* Berkeley, CA: Wilderness Press, 2007.

Blackwell, Laird R. *Wildflowers of the Sierra Nevada and the Central Valley.* Auburn, WA: Lone Pine Publishing USA, 1999.

Blehm, Eric. *The Last Season.* New York: Harper Collins, 2006.

Brewer, William Henry, William H. Alsup, and Yosemite Association. *Such a Landscape!: A Narrative of the 1864 California Geological Survey Exploration of Yosemite, Sequoia & Kings Canyon from the Diary, Field Notes, Letters & Reports of William Henry Brewer.* El Portal, CA: Yosemite Association, 1999.

Browning, Peter. *Sierra Nevada Place Names: From Abbot to Zumwalt,* 3rd edition. Lafayette, CA: Great West Books, 2011.

Clelland, Mike. *Ultralight Backpackin' Tips.* Guilford, CT: Falcon Guides, 2011.

Farquhar, Francis Peloubet. *History of the Sierra Nevada.* Berkeley, CA: University of California Press, 2007.

Gaines, David. *Birds of Yosemite and the East Slope.* Lee Vining, CA: Artemisia Press, 1992.

Ghiglieri, Michael Patrick, and Charles R. "Butch" Farabee Jr. *Off the Wall: Death in Yosemite : Gripping Accounts of All Known Fatal Mishaps in America's First Protected Land of Scenic Wonders.* Flagstaff, AZ: Puma Press, 2007.

Glazner, Allen F., and Greg M. Stock. *Geology Underfoot in Yosemite National Park.* Missoula, MT: Mountain Press Publishing Company, 2010.

Guyton, Bill. *Glaciers of California: Modern Glaciers, Ice Age Glaciers, Origin of Yosemite Valley, and a Glacier Tour in the Sierra Nevada.* Berkeley, CA: University of California Press, 2001.

Horn, Elizabeth L. *Sierra Nevada Wildflowers.* Missoula, MT: Mountain Press Publishing Company, 1998.

Huber, N. King, and Wymond W. Eckhardt. "Devils Postpile Story." Three Rivers, CA: Sequoia Natural History Association, 2001.

Johnston, V. R. *Sierra Nevada—The Naturalist's Companion.* Berkeley, CA: University of California Press, 2000.

King, Clarence. *Mountaineering in the Sierra Nevada.* Lincoln, NE: University of Nebraska Press, 1997.

Laws, John Muir. *The Laws Field Guide to the Sierra Nevada.* Berkeley, CA: Heyday Books, 2007.

Moore, James Gregory. *Exploring the Highest Sierra.* Stanford, CA: Stanford University Press, 2000.

Morey, Kathy, Mike White, Stacy Corless, and Thomas Winnett. *Sierra North,* 9th edition. Berkeley, CA: Wilderness Press, 2005.

Morey, Kathy, Mike White, et al. *Sierra South,* 8th edition. Berkeley, CA: Wilderness Press, 2006.

Roberts, Suzanne. *Almost Somewhere: Twenty-Eight Days on the John Muir Trail.* Lincoln, NE: University of Nebraska Press, 2012.

Roper, Steve. *The Climber's Guide to the High Sierra.* San Francisco: Sierra Club Books, 1976.

Roth, Hal. *Pathway in the Sky.* Berkeley, CA: Howell-North Books, 1965.

Sargent, Shirley. *Solomons of the Sierra: The Pioneer of the John Muir Trail.* Yosemite, CA: Flying Spur Press, 1989.

Secor, R. J. *The High Sierra: Peaks, Passes, and Trails,* 3rd edition. Seattle: The Mountaineers Books, 2009.

Sibley, David. *The Sibley Field Guide to Birds of Western North America.* New York: Knopf, 2003.

Storer, Tracy Irwin, Robert Leslie Usinger, and David Lukas. *Sierra Nevada Natural History.* Berkeley, CA: University of California Press, 2004.

Weeden, Norman. *A Sierra Nevada Flora.* Berkeley, CA: Wilderness Press, 1996.

White, Mike. *Sequoia & Kings Canyon National Parks.* Berkeley, CA: Wilderness Press, 2012.

Wise, James M. *Mount Whitney to Yosemite: The Geology of the John Muir Trail.* Seattle: CreateSpace, 2009.

INDEX

ABOUT THE AUTHOR

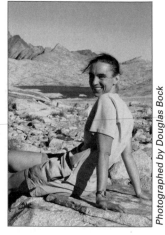

From childhood, **Elizabeth "Lizzy" Wenk** has hiked and climbed in the Sierra Nevada with her family. Since she started college, she has found excuses to spend every summer in the Sierra, with its beguiling landscape, abundant flowers, and near-perfect weather. One interest lies in biological research, and she worked first as a research assistant for others and then completed her own PhD thesis research on the effects of rock type on alpine plant distribution and physiology. However, much of the time, she hikes simply for leisure. Obsessively wanting to explore every bit of the Sierra, she has hiked thousands of on- and off-trail miles and climbed more than 600 peaks in the mountain range. Many of her wanderings are now directed to gather data for several Wilderness Press titles and to introduce her two young daughters to the wonders of the mountains. For them as well, the Sierra, and especially Yosemite, has become a favorite location. Although she will forever consider Bishop, California, home, Wenk is currently living in Sydney, Australia, with her husband, Douglas, and daughters, Eleanor and Sophia. There she is working as a research fellow at Macquarie University and enjoying Australia's exquisite eucalyptus forests, vegetated slot canyons, and wonderful birdlife—except during the Northern Hemisphere summer, which she continues to spend exploring the Sierra.